Illness, My Complicit Enemy

Maria Andreas

Copyright © 2018 Maria Andreas All rights reserved.

Maria Andreas

Illness, My Complicit Enemy

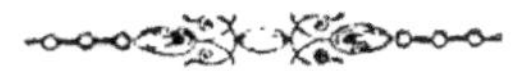

La Maladie, Mon Ennemie Complice

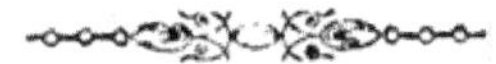

Original French Version, 2018

Translated into English by
Jacqueline Tobin, 2018

Copyright © 2018 Maria Andreas
All rights reserved.

Editions Favrebulle
Biel 2018

Dedication

To Mireille who had the idea for this book.
In memory of her parents, Judith and Laurent.

Contents

Preface

I HAVE THE ENJOYABLE task of writing a few words about this book, a work which illuminates brilliantly the dichotomy that modern medicine seems to have got itself trapped in. Maria Andreas points out, with her characteristic delicacy, the lack of interest that our medicine currently has for listening to the patient, and for how it forgets about the meaningful reality of what it is to be a human with holistic needs. She reminds us, the medical professionals, that in our practice we are dealing with neither a disembodied psyche, nor an inanimate body, but with a complete person ... who has a body that brings with it all its failings and illnesses.

The development of a diagnosis is the result of rational cognitive processes. Having listened to the patient's symptoms, it comes from recognising the combination of signs and confronting them with the knowledge that will allow to us to determine the condition that causes them. But a double reduction takes place during this process: first, the need to filter the patient's speech, to extract what "meets the contingencies provided within the semiology."

The second applies to his or her body, the examination of which will only lead to a diagnosis when the doctor recognises the characteristics of organ suffering. This filtering does not go without its own issues. The patient talks about what is happening to him or her. The lived experience of the illness is present. The patient's subjectivity, his or her rights. As much as we are dealing with an organism, we are dealing with the body's relationships too. Especially with the relationship to the doctor who listens to, speaks to, touches, alerts and soothes him or her. Now we are in the realm of the essential: that of paying attention to the sick person. The patient appears there as a: "subject capable of expression and self-reflection only through possessives: his or her pain and how they represent it, their anguish, their hopes and dreams."[1]

Maria Andreas has the lucidity and the courage to announce that: illness has something to teach us!

Through her expertise as a patient, through her story, Maria Andreas makes us think of a medical approach that exists between Earth and Heaven, like a band of Möbius, and allows us to draw back together that which a dualistic conception came to disjoin and what we have got used to thinking of as oppositions: science versus art, technical versus relationships, certified knowledge versus accumulated experience, cure and care, the treatment of illness and the treatment of the sick.

I am certain that the lesson to be discovered through this work, a work that is well-illustrated and remarkably well-argued, will be regarding the importance of reconciling these two aspects and thereby linking their twinned potential.

Doctor Gérard Ostermann
Professor of Therapeutics, Internist and French Psychotherapist-Analyst

[1] G. Canguilhem, *Étude D'histoire Et De Philosophie Des Sciences*, Vrin, Paris, 1983

Foreword

Illness…
An enemy to flush out, to annihilate by all means!
And yet, illness can also become … "an accomplice"!
To discover that my projects, my will, my intelligence can capsize, at the very second of a medical verdict, a fall, an accident. I am not, as I had thought, the master of my destiny … And perhaps, through this imposed suffering, I will approach another form of intelligence, of will, of destiny … escaping the proud routine of my confinement, of my egoism … to welcome … the other … and …
Why not … The Other?

Prologue

This book describes A daily struggle, that has become a way of life, since I have gone through numerous illnesses, surgical operations and tough ordeals.

There's nothing original about that! That's why I begin by putting everyone, anyone who has lived, or is living through, these kinds of experience, on guard.

And ... that is equally true of this book!

Our somatic and psychological traumas, if they register themselves both in statistics and in everyday medical practice, remain unique. This must lead everyone to develop their own battle plan, as well as their own specific "complicity" with the ordeal. These multiple tactics can then meet, share, fertilise each other. As long as they agree to withdraw, faced with the uniqueness of the Person and the other's path.

My life experience will never be ... your life experience!

My advice is to check for yourselves!

That's why the answers not there in the Google search results. Everything is *experienced*! My wish, with this book, is to stimulate those who are going through trials. Which, of course, will offer similarities to those I have gone through. For other readers, it would be a great reward, if this book prompted some preventative measures!

But above all, I hope that this book will incite some searching ... delving around, in and around oneself, for what will become one's battlefield ... of conquests ... and ... of victories!

Of course, this book is not a substitute for advice and medical opinion.

I continue to express my gratitude to Science and to all the medical staff, who allowed me to have the strength and the life to write this testimony.

"Death, My Little Sister?"

IT WAS MY THERAPIST in Bordeaux, who, one day, pronounced, this sentence...

It stayed with me ... Undoubtedly because I will never reach this conviviality with Death ...

Yet Death was very present ... even before my birth.

My parents, living in Kenya, had no wish yet for a child. Mum, who had been uprooted from the high school where she excelled, to be a vendor at the age of 15, was training as a secretary. The previous embryos, fruits of the passionate tropical nights of this couple who adored each other body and soul, had been entrusted to the care of the British abortionist ...

Blow of Destiny ... the facetiousness of Life?

When it was my turn ...

The abortionist was on holiday!

So, the young couple in love concluded that they were happy to start a family sooner than expected!

Not wanting to expose the life of their future baby to the perils that preceded decolonisation, my parents abandoned their earthly paradise, to land in Algiers. This is where I saw the light ... and the sea for the first time.

The sea ... a miracle that I will always be asking for during my future convalescences.

Forceps birth, followed by a transient "amnesia", because upon being revived Mum did not recognise the father, her beloved, nor the piece of flesh that was presented to her and which had a lemon colour ...

It was the famous jaundice of newborns, which was treated with spoonfuls of Vichy water.

Having abandoned everything in Kenya, the young parents were left broke in a city where apartments were scarce.

It was in the garden of a modest ground floor apartment that Death tried her luck a second time. I had been allowed to sleep in the garden: the fresh air having featured largely in my life to strengthen me, right from birth. I was crying, as regularly reported by the neighbours' adorable little boy. No doubt that day, more strongly than usual ...

When my parents came back, they found in my cradle a big paving slab next to my head, ... just on the wrong side ...

Or rather ... seen from my side ... just on the right side!

We moved to the 7th, with a terrace, where I could, at my leisure, compete with the songs of the neighbouring minaret ...

At two years old, I could already express myself well, but I wasn't walking.

When consulted, the paediatrician in his fifties decreed that I was perfectly normal, since I was speaking!

A second time decolonisation drove us away ...

Back home, my paternal grandmother patiently stood me on my legs every day. Until I could keep pace with my little cousins, who looked suspiciously at this runt, (so close to having been aborted in fact), half tropical, half black feet.

Starting out again from zero, the couple, still in love, gave me the present of a jewel of a little brother.

There were errors of course! Especially the psychological ones! Tragic sometimes, like those who forever derailed my younger brother's life, who in addition suffered from a genetic disease…discovered… when he was 60 years old.

Ignorance, the worst of enemies!

Accursèd Ignorance!

I open a parenthesis, to say to all parents, that the first, not to say the only gift, that they can ever offer to their children, is that of their own "maturing". And work, which they first accepted on their own, regardless of their family and social background. I would add banality to this, and that also applies to love-relationships, or any other deep human relationship.

But we do not go back! Our parents, children of the Crash years of '29, one having grown up in an apocalyptic sect, the other with an unbalanced mother, cherished us. They did their best to make us "strong".

Spiritually, I would say that their permanent quest allowed me to meet, at a very young age, many so-called "esoteric" circles of the time. As for my paternal grandparents, whom I loved, their Christian faith was, alas, mostly based on fear and divine punishment. But their intention was so pure that they knew how to transmit a taste for prayer to me ...

If I make a comparison with the average way of life today, I would say that we were raised healthily.

Quasi-vegetarian food, black bread, lots of fruits and vegetables, dairy products and ... the great outdoors, the great outdoors, the great outdoors.

Sport too. Lots of sport.

My favourite was swimming.

Although I foolishly just avoided drowning myself at the age of 12 (by venturing into the raging sea during a storm), I only felt good in the water ...

Dad and my brother were veritable ski champions!

What a shame for me, who never failed to sprain my ankle as soon as I strapped these planks, that I always judged to be disproportionate, to my feet!

Peritonitis, operated upon urgently, introduced me for the first time to the hospital environment.

But overall, my childhood, thanks to parental vigilance, rolled along pretty nicely.

Well enough in any case for me to approach adolescence with the great project of freeing myself from the "health constraints" of the house.

By the time I was 15, I was smoking like a big shot and the daily pack of cigarettes quickly replaced the great outdoors. Worse still, it escorted it at the top of its lungs!

At 20, I granted myself cocktails, the contraceptive pill and tobacco!

Smoking more and more, despite repeated angina ...

After my studies, answering the call of hippies of the time, I embarked with my companion, in a VW bus in the direction of Asia, then North Africa. Our main delicacies consisted of packets of soup and jam. But, I was in the open air, often I was swimming in the sea ... and I was feasting on life!

A stay in Cambridge, to get my teaching certificate and to continue ... to eat the world ... smoking ...

On my return, I entered a renowned private institute as a languages teacher, in the German part of Switzerland.

Half hippie in the 70s, still lulled by recent British phlegm, I was forced to make an immediate review of myself, heart and soul!

The director, at the head of the establishment, undertook to re-educate me! By the way, I would advise young people never to slam the door, when an experienced senior does not find them quite as great as they imagined ...

This man taught me my job ... and more: he taught me to fight!

According to one of his famous phrases (they are all engraved in my memory 40 years later!):

"Problems are there to be solved! "

Naturally, he never hindered my freedom ... and richer and just as free, I continued to smoke.

Yes, yes, I see myself in the middle of winter, after each class, (we had 28 to 32 of them per week in a full-time post), rushing into the icy courtyard, to light a cigarette, without disturbing colleagues in the staffroom!

I continued to feast on life, because I loved my job!

Too much, doubtless, in the eyes of my companion who,

prey to the worst of passions, jealousy, made my evenings and weekends a real hell.

I have no wish to tell here of the traumatic events. Since then they have been forgiven or even assimilated. From the great height of my splendid 28 years, I certainly ignored his suffering. In simple terms, I wonder why we stay living in unsustainable situations, the ending of which we cannot ignore. There exists a kind of paralysis, a morbidity in certain states of immobility. As if we had to ... atone ...

Atone…

Yes, sometimes, when I think about it or think of certain relatives who have gone through this form of Hades, no other word comes to me than that of atonement ... Is it a part of The Way?

It was at that time of violent daily quarrels, that Death, for the fourth time, approached ...

"The best way to win," I was advised by the one we named "The Leader," was to always return to my classes! He was right! This endless return literally welded me to my workplace ...

Rough times though! Nerves on edge ... but ... I continued to adore my job, to smoke more than ever ... to eat ... and ... life ... and ... everything that calmed me down. Mainly sweets, pastries, fries ... in considerable quantity ...

In order to keep to my dress size, I embarked on diets, as aberrant as they were excessive, during the holidays ...

It was exactly then that my spine manifested itself for the first time.

There were pains, a stiff back, but nothing that really disturbed my consciousness.

I felt young and ... healthy!

Mocking the doctor, who claimed that my spine was three times my age!

Helped by the smoking, I also began to develop year-round bronchitis.

I still see the bottles of *Famel* syrup that the leader slipped into my locker.

A disgusting taste of petrol ... but it helped me to stay on my feet ...

Quickly however, it was necessary to move on to a tougher plan! First of all for my back which had two injections a year, (the maximum dose that we set for my thirties), cocktails of cortisone and *Voltarene*. The latter can also be taken orally, by means of some negotiations with my stomach. As for my bronchi, diagnosed tightened and affected, they began a long relationship with antibiotics. Associated themselves with cortisone sprays. This last teaching term does not arouse the least suspicion in my heart ... I continued to eat life and ... this wonderful job!

Astonishing, but true, it was a time when we only missed our lessons when we were at Death's door.

And that did not shock us. I would even add ... that sometimes it "healed" us!

It should be noted that no union group haunted these hard-working places that were proud to be so!

My colleagues were practically all from the opposite sex. This did not altogether displease me. I liked their frank way of talking, that was sometimes rude, even at my own expense. I adapted my language to theirs, and I followed them as best as I could. This was how I found myself in this Piper[2], for a memorable flight destined to put a stop to my fear of planes. It was into this little Piper, as moving as it was comical, that Death tried to slip herself for the fifth time ... The college gymnastics teacher, a friendly daredevil, made me climb into the front. And ... "Baptism by Piper" requires, he realised, according to what was customary, many antics taking photos, all while filling the tank.

While taking off, I was surprised to breathe in a strong smell of fuel. I yelled at him: "It stinks of gas!"

"No problem! Look how beautiful it is! We will soon be

---

[2] Light aircraft, one-engined, built in 1927

flying over the Institute!" But suddenly ... he put both his hands on my shoulders and shouted as calmly as courageously,

"Don't worry, we'll have a beautiful landing!"

The airfield was already far behind us and the Institute was still far ahead of us ... I understood ... and ... I also understood what "shitting your pants" meant!

He had failed to close the fuel tank!

She didn't have ... me ... she ... didn't have ... us... !

Death!

Just a few good shakes, in a freshly-cut a field of wheat ...

Indeed ... the daredevil ... made a beautiful landing!

I had an unexpected reaction ...

Hardly had the door of the plane opened, than I rushed headlong into this wheat field and, atheist that I was, laughed sobbingly: "Thank you my God, thank you! "

Convinced that life still wanted me, I decided to eat even more of it. For every day of the holiday, there was a travel plan! But at barely 30, my body's frame began to rebel cruelly against this! My circulatory issues were revealed when I bit into some varicose veins between two courses. Backache intensified. Bronchitis was almost year-round.

At 30, alarm bells finally managed to alert my logical side. I decided to throw away my pack of cigarettes from that day onwards! I managed the feat of not going back to them, with a weight gain of ten kilos! I overcame this surplus weight, eating appetite suppressants, that were banned from the market soon afterwards ...

One day, a friend introduced me to a doctor, stricken from the medical register for methods considered dangerous ... Yet ... I gave him my jugular vein, in which he regularly planted needles. Injecting me with various products of his own making ...

In vain ... bronchitis took hold ...

My coughing could be heard from one end of the college to the other ...

But I still loved my job as much as ever, and I still ate life up ... however, it began to eat me too ...

It was more and more difficult recuperating during the holidays ...

As for outings, in 25 years, I have strictly performed only those "prescribed" for the accompanying of my students to theatres, concerts or the cinema.

Little by little, a chronic fatigue became a partner to my respiratory troubles. I made up for it with long nights, holidays that were focused more and more on seaside stays, sources of regeneration. During the school year, it was with a litre of cola a day, and an abundance of chocolate and coffee.

To add to my bronchitis, there was a collection of repeated bouts of cystitis ... long live antibiotics!

That did not prevent me, after a conversion to orthodoxy, from taking theology correspondence courses, in a Parisian institute, where ... I even married one of my teachers!

The latter, on a professional mission, settled in Aix-en-Provence.

Not wanting to abandon my institute, I undertook to reshape my life: holidays in the South, as well as two weekends a month! This amounted to doing nine hours of train journeys on Friday afternoons and nine more on Sunday nights ... Sleeping cars being an assured source of microbes and viruses, I multiplied infections of all kinds ... Long live antibiotics!

My desire to have a child, for different reasons, had no results. So, more than ever, I clung to my job. Raised in an environment where psychotherapy was excluded from our morals, it didn't occur to me at that time, the idea never came, to dig a little, which was a suffering...

One day, I remember very well, I was in Zurich, early October '89. I was looking for a baptismal dress for my niece and godchild. It was mild and I loved to walk in this city. Yet after an hour, I felt unusually tired and began to sweat profusely. I don't know why, but a spark flashed across my mind, with the warning: "You, my daughter, you're breeding a bitch in there"... A bitch we will call it 16 years later ...

In the meantime, I had joint pains, and a constant fever. And excessive exhaustion became my permanent companion.

Medical visits and all-round checks! In 1991, a laparoscopy detected a large myoma in my womb. I remember most of all, that it is anaesthesia that I have coped least well with in my life. Fixed up with eight hot-water bottles and an army of blankets in my bed, I kept shivering until I hurt horribly all the night through. This unremarkable little examination had also exhausted me. I can see my brother now, searching for me at the hospital and saying, "It's not a hospital discharge, it's an abduction!" so exhausted was I ...

In 1992 we removed everything, the myoma and the womb ... Operation during the spring break. Success, convalescence ... and ... despair ... because the fever was still there. A doctor-friend suggested that it was alarming and could become a breeding-ground for cancer ... I didn't even register this reference ...

But this job that I loved, turned into a cross ... Weakening, ruined immune system, bronchitis, pneumonia, viruses of all kinds, cystitis, angina ... and I could go on ...

Regularly, I brought my guts up. Probably intestinal viruses, because even today, these are the ones that I catch the fastest and fear the most!

A doctor-friend, passing by during a session of vomiting, suggested upon its palpation that my liver was too big. He wasn't listened to!

In April 1996, about forty varicose veins and my two lateral saphenous veins were removed ...

In July, exhausted, I surrender ... and I re-join my husband, who has just retired to Bordeaux.

Determined to rest ...

But ... not forever.

I spend a long quiet summer and enrol at the University of Classical Letters in September!

My enthusiasm for the Greek language is vibrant ... but I'm

still so exhausted ...

Assuming depression, due to the loss of my job, I decide to undertake psychotherapy.

I am looking back on myself that first time, sitting in what is undoubtedly the best office in Bordeaux, in front of my therapist who - God be blessed - had also been trained as an internist doctor.

What grace!

He agrees to give me the therapy, but finds that I have a complexion which he describes as "hepatic".

Bingo ...

But, once again, she did not get me!

Analyses reveal the hepatitis C virus. So *voilà*, the bitch finally has a name!

Another grace: the RNA is negative, which means that the virus is relenting, or better still, that it has been defeated!

Having knowledge around me, which wasn't really the case, my gratitude was overflowing ... and ... I finally attacked myself with a serious regime, which I will describe later.

However, I did not go back to university ...

In 1999, despite not knowing anyone there we have decided to spend a year in Cyprus. Our desire is to learn the language, culture and especially to open up the vault of orthodoxy.

But at what cost! Monstrous summer heatwave very poorly dealt with ... in a more than spartan studio! At the first cold winds of November, I found myself almost stuck fast in the street! Fearing a serious worsening of my lumbar and cervical hernias, I stayed lying down ... then ... January 2000, with a heavy heart, despite our more than ascetic lifestyle, we came back to a huge bill ...

However, I want to open a parenthesis:

Cyprus, Greece and the Byzantine world, have allowed us to discover the treasure for which we have been looking for a long time. Not because we had acquired for ourselves a stashed address from a spiritual haven! Nor because parents or friends had emigrated and we wanted to be in the sun ourselves! But ...

because the treasures are rare ... very rare. They can only be caught at the price of ... I drop in this word, which hasn't been kind to me, so far: "suffering".

On the way back, I can still hear the rheumatologist: "There is good news and bad news: the good news: it's not your back ... the bad news, your dysplastic right hip is completely worn and it's too late to intervene ... except ... with a total replacement! "

Cripes ... I'm not yet 50 years old ... But now the mystery of my delayed walking is cleared up ... Congenital hip dysplasia ... Head of the femur too small and completely worn ...

A whole year ... a year of visits, physiotherapy, reflections ... The medical body is almost unanimous: the more we push the positioning of the prosthetic in, the better ... and here I am wearing two crutches ... from January 2000 to April 2003! My deep commitment to independence takes a hit on the nose ... Fortunately I am accompanied well ... because when shopping on two crutches, only ideal for straight lines ... you don't buy too many potatoes!

Is it the hassle, annoyance? But at this time an arrhythmia, hitherto disdained by me, annoys me more and more ... A few years later, the detection of a small congenital leak of the mitral valve will place me under *Flecaine,* which I still take to this day.

Nevertheless, I enrol myself in Greek classes at university and, armed with crutches, I pass my first year exams.

In 2001, however, I am offered a consultation with a renowned orthopaedic surgeon in Zurich. His verdict is uncompromising! Operate on my hip dysplasia as soon as possible. To my question about my "precocious" age for this kind of intervention, he retorts: "You're screwing up your spine with these crutches! Besides ... do you know if you'll still be here in ten years?" Shaken by this realist insolence, I ask him, since he is about to retire, who his collaborators are. Resolved to keep the first name he writes down ...

That's when I come home ... to Switzerland. This Switzerland that will become, in my "gypsy globe-trotting" heart, *My Switzerland!*

A small country that does not only consist of banks and money! But also of a hardworking, courageous people ... which reassures me ...

2002, March 3, our uncle dies of cancer. I remember perfectly the conversation with his daughter-in-law, who tells me, "What I'm afraid of is breast cancer!"

"Ah yes, exactly, I have my mammogram tomorrow!" Undergoing hormone replacement since 1995, I have a regular check-up every two years. Each time, with a light heart, having no family history and not feeling at all concerned ...

I will come back to prevention later, but I open a parenthesis to praise, bless and recommend mammograms!

Bang in the middle: it's my turn!

Stunned, the left breast petrified by a dozen additional mammos, I call an old friend, the doctor from Zurich, who advises me on the best surgeon.

This best or, at least in 2002, one of the best, accompanied me for many years.

Again, I see him now after the biopsy, telling me, while I was lying down, about the discovery of two separate and very aggressive tumours! He approached me, traced a curve just above the nipple and whispered, "The safest thing would be amputation! And ... I have the nerve to retort:

"Doctor, I would like to fight for my breast!"

During the next two weeks, while he's consulting with the biologist, the pathologist, the oncologist and the radiologist, I realise that what really matters to me is to survive ... and I'm ready for anything!

I believe that my faithful companions, the crutches, were of this opinion... My husband too, untiring companion in this journey across Hades...

Finally, the best, with the agreement of his colleagues,

decides upon a conservative operation, followed by 50 sessions of radiotherapy.

The best has really accomplished something! He has taken a quarter of my left breast ... and nobody will see anything at all! Finally, there is nothing at all to be seen because after the operation and then the x-rays, it's *bonjour* to the grilling!

Left ganglia removed, (complete axillary lymphadenectomy). It only remains for me to wait for the biopsy ... but he lets me know that I will see the oncologist soon ...

I still remember his lovely assistant, that 23rd April 2002, St George's Day, approaching my bed smiling. She gives me the report ...

"Is it good?"

She smiled again, "yes!"

Aggressive tumours ... but ... no metastasis!

I whisper, "blessed be medicine! "

She goes on, "and blessed be those who get tested early! "

The professor decides that I won't have chemo, although opinions are not unanimous.

The second champion, the great professor of radiology, his friend, receives me a few weeks later for the x-rays.

Tumours are receptive to hormones, they put me under Tamoxifen. He explains to me ... and I see him now, on a sweet May morning - that this kind of cancer can, on the one hand, return locally. Hence the need to go under the grill! On the other hand, it could spread in about ten years, although treatment reduces this risk.

At this moment, as I write these lines, it has already been 16 years ...

Tomorrow maybe? After tomorrow? In a year? In 10 years ...

Never ...

God only knows! In any case, as I describe later, I do everything in my power to prevent a recurrence ...

In the meantime, I reward myself with a frozen shoulder[3], during the first x-ray session. My barely healed underarm gives me the feeling of being torn (which isn't the case) and for each of the 50 sessions, raising my arm above my head, is torture ...

Neither is it that great to press down on crutches with a frozen shoulder...

The best, the one who never gives in to pessimism, promises me that with regular physiotherapy and especially swimming, I will recover use of my shoulder. The excellent physiotherapist, to whom he entrusts me for months, will confess to me later that when she saw me, she had thought that my shoulder would never recover!

The best, him again, suggests to me that the immobility my crutches impose on me, harms my general state. To move is an indispensable reflex, after cancer ... He advises me ... another 'best', to have an operation on my hip ... On none other than the one that I'd retained, during my visit in 2001...

Eight months after cancer, I find myself on the operating table again, for a total hip replacement.

Perfect orthopaedic success! Leg length adjusted, a screw in the pelvis and hoops around the femur, to reinforce its strength in the face of osteopenia.

But my whole body's frame is crushed ...

Exhausted ...

Haggard ...

And the pains are tenacious ... Not at all from my new hip ... no, from my back ... Stretched out, without any opportunity to turn around, with a big "cheese" between my thighs, to keep me from crossing my legs, I'm immersed in pain day after day ... night after night ...

Is my back jealous of this beautiful operation?

In any case, after six weeks, it wasn't complaining about no longer being welded to crutches! What a liberation ... Even if

---

[3] Today, with new techniques for the removal of sentinel lymph nodes, there is less risk of a frozen shoulder.

going up slopes is a slow business ...

I won, by dint of patience ... of physio ... despite my still-frozen shoulder, and despite my hip in rehabilitation. One day, my health insurance summons me to call them. They wanted to know why I was seeing two physiotherapists, sometimes both on the same day. I replied: "one's for my shoulder, the other's for my hip! "

By the end of 2003, I found my shoulder capacity was 100%! And…

I had been walking without crutches and without pain since April.

In the spring of 2004, during my first trip abroad with a patched-up skeleton, I once again had a brush with Death. Through being poisoning, according to later research, by contaminated tap water. Never in my life had I vomited so much, nor suffered so much evil in every millimetre of my body. Never before, either, had I experienced this "black veil" across my eyes and my head in flames. One wall of my stomach stuck to the other, I really thought it was the end. Brought to the emergency room by ambulance, I stayed under observation that night and the next day. Nothing abnormal there ... if I may say so ... However, with anti-emetics I remained in my bed for ten days, exhausted. I did not recover until I was finally able to dive into the sea!

Since then, when travelling abroad I drink only bottled water, boiled water or with *Micropur Forte* pellets!

Upon return, the only thing that remained was ... to continue with the battle! A battle against infections, with a deficient immune system.

It's because of this that I'm interested in everything, everything that I'll describe in this book.

I say that forcefully, because the aggravation of my back pain was ... almost unavoidable ...

I remember the great professor's slip up in 2003, after a thorough consultation including the whole of my spine and cervical hernias: "At the top it's not as dramatic ... I mean ... it's not as serious as what's at the base…"

Since 2008, it's hell and only those who know the torture of the spine, know what I'm talking about. At the end of 2008, I take back the crutches... and the whole panoply for delaying the operation (injections etc...) is put into place.

In November 2009, the professor told me, "we will get rid of these crutches!"

Grafts, artificial discs, splayed channels, fasteners with screws and plates... the whole package!

I see him again, after five hours of Great Leader's work, in the intensive care room, pinching my fingers and toes and noting the result.

Once again ... Once again ... Once again!

Four months later, I am released, I am walking ... and the battle is resumed!

I'm 60 years old...

But family constraints hinder my plans for a somatic redesign and healthy living ... I do *minium* physio, with one of the queens of physio. I try to rest, to live as healthily as possible and to do this often. But years of fatigue weigh heavily and grow the list of infections, especially in the lungs. The most virulent, in January 2015, will be worth an extended stay in hospital. All possible research on metastases will be done by the oncologist - a top champion - who has been following me quarterly since 2003.

Nothing ... Nada ... Rien … Nichts ... Tipota!

Praise God ... We continue!

I no longer have the audacity, nor the insolence to make calculations, nor to add that, once again, Death did not have me ...

In the meantime, she took away my younger and only brother, in August 2016, with leukaemia ...

And then… this April 29, 2018, on taking up my pen, I must unfortunately add two "stars" to my list of prize-winners. In December 2017, I caught aggressive bronchitis that had the "merit" of revealing a background of asthma. Those who suffer from asthmatic bronchitis know just how much filamentous sputum clings. Full of cough, it was during an effort to clear it, involving a degree of torsion, that I broke a vertebra (L1). This has revealed osteoporosis of the spine (which cannot be measured if you have scrap metal in your bones). One thing to be thankful for however, the doctor assured me, was that this fracture was not caused by any bone metastases. After six weeks of intensive pain, my back was re-operated on, January 23, 2018, by the same champion as in 2009. A successful kyphoplasty! But … I had to start my rehabilitation from scratch! With a weakened back and shock that I have yet to get over.

The torsion, however, gave me the opportunity to think! To try to discern what was crooked in me … and around me! And then, it had the advantage of pointing out the danger of osteoporosis on my spine, which has since been treated with an annual *Aclasta* injections. Taking care, finally, not to neglect my calcium intake.

But…

The fight remains a mystery …

Healing – how one does it - also remains a mystery …

Loving life, loving your own life, is perhaps one of the components of it … but by far and away not the only one!

And every psycho-emotional digression about failed attempts at healing, except from confirmed and devoted experts in this field, will always seem to me to be as monstrous as it are stuffed full of sterile pride!

Who are you to comment on the suffering, illness or death of another? Under the pretext that you read Jung, Jacques Salomé or that you pray?

Voilà…

In broad outline, I give you here the diary of my ailments … To those that I could hurt in listing them, even in my lightest of tones, I ask for pardon. And I apologise to the reader for bothering him or her with these autobiographical details.

The fact is, they are all, absolutely … faithfully, autobiographical!

And their story has no other purpose than that of truth. With the hope that they will arouse in others a taste for prevention ...

Prevention, this is where the little miracle begins!

The tips I will try to convey have all, without exception, been applied to my life. For the most part, they still are. In this new life, afforded to me by God, science, and those wonderful men and women who have dedicated their lives to it.

In this regard, I naturally wish to thank my Creator ...

And all those who carried me in their prayers!

The one, who physically by my side, carried me ... simple as that!

But also the doctors, who have enabled me to testify today. I thought of listing them one by one. I hope they'll forgive me, but on the one hand, it would be too long, and on the other, it would risk giving those who will be operated on in the future, the feeling that they may not have a good surgeon. However, if you are reading these lines and are concerned about one illness or another, I advise you to fight hard to find *the partner* ... Yes, yes, it is about a partner who has given over so many years of his or her youth to study, and who will look into your case! Trust is essential. It searches for itself ... and it creates itself. As a Christian, I always prayed for my doctors, before their interventions. I continue to do it afterwards ... and every day at that. If you are not religious, then send him or her your good thoughts, your trusting energies, before they cut into you. And above all, never launch into the stupid idea that he or she earns too much ... while you are not indignant about the so much higher salary of the boy you admire, running behind a ball, or screaming into a microphone!

And then, you have to put this in your head: as good as he or she is, your doctor will never be able to do your physio for you, or take your medication, or adapt your lifestyle and triumph on your behalf!

All healing begins, or at least continues, when you close the door to the doctor's room. It will always be a synergy ... a partnership!

We are not married to our 'quacks' either, even if some of

them are very good-looking! And sometimes, it is essential to ask for a second opinion. Make that change if the partnership doesn't work anymore! Our generation has the privilege of being able to learn things on the Internet, to exchange with other patients on the web. But we must digest, verify, discern, because sometimes the opposite effect is achieved. It may worry you needlessly or set you off on the wrong track!

Also park the *illuminated*, the decision-makers! Though I had the chance to meet excellent homeopaths (the last, just recently, just before his retirement) and herbal therapists, to complement my treatments, I remember landing myself in a doctor's room, where I was ordered to stop any treatment for cancer immediately!

Having crossed paths with them, I lost two dear friends to these kinds of dangers ...

No, I do not question miracles of nature, nor miracles full stop ...

But we have to admit, they are not as frequent as we would like!

Of course, there are also, and more and more so, doctors and hospitals interested in complementary approaches that were considered heretical a few years ago. Chinese medicine, sophrology, reflexology, even magnetism, hypnosis etc ... and as far as it speaks to you, you would be really wrong not to give it a go. A great surgeon or oncologist does not have time to become familiar with those methods. So it's up to you to search, to strike, and to test it out!

Yes, try, regardless of various comments, because as can never be repeated enough: we are all different!

What follows has helped me a lot ... and continues to help me.

I express the wish that this may serve to alert, and if possible prevent. To maybe lay down some tracks to help manage all this damage that our bodies go through during our lives.

I will start with:

Osteoarthritis

Although there were other causes of congenital deformities, the three operations that I underwent, first on my hip, then on my spine, were largely to repair the damage caused by osteoarthritis.

If you want to try to calm and halt the progression of your osteoarthritis (because we cannot cure it), there is good news and bad news. The bad news will always be the same: it takes investment, consistency and discipline. Sometimes having to deprive yourself of what you consider to be your joys and a part of your freedom. And rightly, think about your freedom. Osteoarthritis is one of your worst enemies. Of your freedom of movement and independence in any case!

The good thing is that by following certain rules on a regular basis, (one can never boast enough about regularity!), you will kill two birds with one stone! You will be giving a facelift to your arteries, your cardiovascular system and your pump! Even more, since inflammation is a welcoming nest for cancer, you will help your body to strengthen itself.

The great enemy of osteoarthritis is easily imagined – being overweight... and lack of movement. Yes, we think that with osteoarthritis we must economise on movement to save ourselves and quite the contrary is true!

As for inflammation (which worsens osteoarthritis pain), it loves butter, dairy products and red meats!

So we have to limit them and, during flare ups, do without them.

Similarly, with ... as you may well suspect: alcohol!

And ... to extend the list of forbidden pleasures, cola and sweets are, as applies to so many evils, to be avoided as much as possible.

As for barbecues, all fried food raises the rate of what is called glycation[4]. And too high a level risks - among other mischiefs - increasing inflammation. When talking about helping

---

[4] The complex binding of sugars with proteins. A biochemical reaction responsible for aging and various harmful bodily complications.

your heart, avoiding or at least reducing them, promotes good cardiovascular function. Moreover, according to some scientists it seems that there is a link between cardiovascular disease, high rates of blood clotting and osteoarthritis.

On the other hand, long live nuts; almonds; berries and currants; spices such as ginger and turmeric. The effectiveness of the latter increases by 1000%, if it is mixed with black pepper. I take a little pot of mustard, I add a teaspoon of black pepper and a soup spoon of turmeric, olive oil (important) and I mix. Sometimes I improve my sauce with yoghurt. (Excellent with a slice of chicken.) And now that fresh turmeric is even found in the supermarket, I cut a piece and boil it for ten minutes, then I drink it. I must say, however, that during irritations of the stomach, I avoid my rations of turmeric. Also long live olive and rapeseed oils; red peppers; cabbages (I digest them better in the evening); cinnamon that will transform your tasteless natural soy yogurt (add it at will); goji berries; cherries and cherry juice; grapes; chestnuts; fennel seeds; oily fish (sardines, mackerel, herring, salmon); and Omega 3.

And ... garlic! We will talk about it again, this blessed garlic, for cancer! (In any case, whatever you adopt from what has been written above is, as I mentioned, part of the anti-cancer diet.)

In homeopathy, one can take *Radium Bromatum 9CH*, (five granules, three times a day), in the case of a flare up. Always in its natural state: the *harpagophytum* found in capsules. Horsetail also. Still *au naturel*, in the case of flare ups, rub in the *Consoude* ointment of our grandmothers!

Regarding grandmothers, something that mine used against acidity, one of the rare things that I cannot stand: clay. She would lay a teaspoon of clay in a glass of water at night. On an empty stomach, she swallowed it without flinching.

I tested the famous green mussel powder. I don't cope with it very well, especially during hot weather, when the smell becomes ruthless.

Disappointing to me as well, was the famous shark cartilage, however, it does suit many.

On the other hand, I often come back to my *Chondroitin-Glucosamine* cures. It seems that the proof is scientifically established, not that it heals osteoarthritis, but halts it ... unless it's in your spine!

You should also ensure that your posture is correct. If not, you'll need orthopaedic insoles and it will be *adieu* ballet shoes! Personally, if I separate myself from my insoles for a few weeks, (wearing only sandals for example), my knee pain comes back! But be careful to find an orthopaedic specialist who is very attentive to your specific problem!

There are also special cushions, for a good sitting posture, at the office or in the car.

And then ... banal, and again banal ... but I insist:

Move! Modern society is pushing to repair age and glue it back together. Now, it is well known that everything that's in motion is developing. Whatever is unused atrophies. Professor Froböser (professor at the University of Sport in Cologne), says that by getting the elderly in old people's homes really moving about, some could come back home!

More and more, doctors are underlining that cartilage wears out ... especially when it's not used, because it is not then being irrigated!

Activity that is regular and practised gently ...

Yes, yes, do not dash blindly down a concrete street in your trainers, running behind your dog, or your Jules that you want to impress!

Walk straight, at a pace that suits you, and look how good it is to go forward, being awake to everything you meet ... Jules and the mutt included!

Of course, the most favourable sports for osteoarthritis are those that do not put pressure on your joints, such as cycling and swimming.

For me, swimming is my survival, my cure, my paradise ...

If possible in the open air, if possible in a lake, a river ... or the sea.

The divine ... the sea, the one I loved, from my first breath in Algiers in 1950!

When one has already been operated on, (back and/or hip), as in my case, it is about swimming properly. I put on my flippers, I turn onto my back and start to dance rhythmically, beating my feet and raising one arm after another.

I cannot sing out enough about the miracle of the sea ...

Swim in the sea...

Simply swim, it won't hurt you!

Okay, even at low cost, travelling chips into the budget and often in our latitudes the winter is long. So, in times of crisis, I award myself a mini Dead Sea bath at an unbeatable price. I buy salt from this famous sea and I put a good cup of it, (quantity to be adapted, depending on what you are coping with, but avoid peeling!) into a bucket of warmish water. I soak my wrists and/or my feet. After about 15 minutes, I gently massage them with comfrey cream or *Rumalaya* cream (based on Ayurvedic herbs from India).

Regular physiotherapy is also essential! Which is to say that you find a good physiotherapist who devises a programme especially for you. You work through this programme, not only during the sessions prescribed annually by your specialist but, also, you discipline yourself to follow this programme ... for life ... and on a daily basis. (I take a break on Sunday.) Better a constant routine, than a gust of wind here and there, more harmful than anything else. Not funny huh? Not really, not much! But I'll give you some comfort! You may not become hooked on them, but befriend your sessions. At first you will feel soothing relief at the end of them, including in your head, where the blood will flow better! Then ... whatever your age, your body aesthetics will also benefit ... I won't do you a drawing, but take a picture, six months before and six months after!

Now, during flare ups it's imperative to stop these sports activities. You must completely rest aching joints (walking stick, bed, splints ...). With the right painkillers, because pain doesn't help. Hot or cold compresses, depending on what relieves you. Both are good.

And be careful … after the flare up and the break from it all, we must resume things smoothly. In any case, when you have osteoarthritis, gentleness is *de rigueur*! Balance and patience … The results will not come in a few weeks, even if some improvement is quickly noticed.

I also try to make a few small movements, throughout the day. Do little "turns" in as many joints as possible. This, along with mini little exercises that are all a bit silly, that I do at any time. For example: arms stretched, fists closed, fists against the shoulder and tightened so that the elbow joint stirs. Or lower and raise your extended foot, or do slight rotations, one ankle after another. Also turn your head right and left, but gently. The same thing for the hands, the fingers, several times a day, extending them, folding them, to make them move, and rotate your wrists. Sitting, swinging your leg forward and backward to make the knee move. For the shoulders, make slight rotations with the arms, small circles. At the end of the day, you will have seen almost nothing, but the traffic will have oiled your joints a little. And you will have realised that your body is alive …

Basically that's a programme that relieves me.

Of course, this list is far from exhaustive. This is just putting down tracks, and then everyone has to complete them for themselves. But all that has been listed above, has been tested by the author and for the most part, continues to be applied.

Another Even More Debilitating Condition: Osteoporosis

As already said in the prologue, I owe my last spine operation of January 2018 to it. The one I had on my vertebra, that broke during a violent coughing fit.

It is vital to prevent it. Especially when there comes a day on which you have no choice but to submit to the operation. For an easy-to-understand reason! It will be complicated to screw your vertebrae or to push the stem of a prosthetic into your femur, if your bones are crumbling. Even if new, pre-operative, bone reinforcement techniques now exist. Densitometry (measuring bone density) every two years is an examination with no side effects. It helps to assess the risk. But be careful, if you have already had an operation and if you have metal in your hip or back. It won't be possible to measure your level of bone density. This is what happened to me. In 2004, I entered the area of osteopenia. I followed the five-year treatment of biphosphonates, via quarterly injections (*Bonviva*). By the way, bisphosphonates reduce the risk of bone metastases after breast cancer. I stopped the treatment in 2009 and the readings, (outside the metallic zones), were correct. Except for … my spine, which has a broken vertebra. I must also say that I neglected to take my calcium dose every day. Furthermore, I always took it along with large amounts of green tea and lemon tea: two excellent drinks, but they reduce the absorption of calcium. Now I drink my green tea at least two hours before or after taking calcium. Following this vertebral fracture, I received my first annual *Aclasta* injection. I bore it well, and decided not to be influenced by the blogs describing the possible side effects! These drugs for osteoporosis are sometimes the cause of much questioning, or even scandal, in the media. I will not list them. Here again, it is up to each and everyone to evaluate their own risks with their doctors, and how to remedy them. Of course, if we come to this kind of treatment, it means that calcium and vitamin D dosage must also be controlled or even adjusted regularly. (Blood tests easily detect levels.)

Finally, to ward off osteoporosis too: move, move, move!

Now a word about the surgeries, particularly the ones to which I submitted my hip and spine. Many of these remarks are as valid for the hip operation as for the back.

The Hip (total replacement, right hip, in 2002, age 52 years)

If I indicate the dates of my operations, it is because progress and evolution are very fast. So, it is advisable to learn about the latest techniques.

In itself, hip replacement is a routine operation that has been practiced for decades!

But the routine is more fun when it's your neighbour! As soon as we know we'll be there, it's less amusing ...

For three years I had been getting about on two crutches. When I lived in Bordeaux, the doctors, especially my rheumatologist, told me to postpone the operation until as late as possible. I might say this was lucky, given that I was nursing two mammary tumours! It was better to start treating the cancer, rather than exhausting myself with another operation ...

In all sincerity, I would not say it's a fun party! And for me, it was all the more painful, as I had just finished the breast operations, with the x-rays and treatments. In addition, after three years of crutches, I wasn't in olympic shape.

Yes, that's where you have to start from. Of course, if you're going to be operated on, it's not going to be because you're in good shape. But, make every effort to arrive in the best state possible.

Psychologically too. It doesn't do to evade fear, or to glean soothing words from the ignorant; or, what is more twisted, to obtain a list of operating failures in the field! Accept the fear, the doubt, but each time, push them away ... tenderly ... Without brusqueness, so that they do not return to take revenge!

Perhaps this is the now-or-never moment to tap into the little something inside you that gives you confidence ... Yes, trust Life, trust God if you believe in Him, and in any case, trust to human science!

I will push this provocation of mine still further: "bless", "rejoice in" this new experience! It will enrich you one way or another! It will be the best kick in the teeth for whatever troubles you! And ... you don't have much to lose!

That does not mean that you take it lightly! Prepare yourself as best you can!

The following is from my own experience:

Disagreements:

I'm at home with liver weaknesses, related to the anaesthetic (whatever it was). I foresee one dose of *phosphorus 15 CH* per week, in the morning before breakfast for four weeks after the operation.

It's also found in homeopathy and I took the so-called recommended dose: *before anaesthetic* and another *after anaesthetic.* I swallowed it just before, with the consent of the anaesthetist and I took the one on waking as soon as I could.

Being endowed, as a bonus, with a *dolichocolon* (an extremely long colon, which happens sometimes in women), I am routinely constipated after surgical intervention. But in fact, dolicho or not, that's the fate of most people when they are operated on. Before operations, I ask (if the medical staff don't offer it) to be "gently drained". Before the hip replacement, I enjoyed a good syrup of figs for example. Before the kyphoplasty, I had a gentle enema the day before.

If constipation lasts, glycerin suppositories or even mini enemas can be provided, but in consultation with staff. In the meantime, during the first days, homeopathy offers several remedies against the inevitable gases. If it really stinks, when your gorgeous surgeon visits you, you can take three granules of *Kalium Carbonicum 5CH* before main meals.

I also took, five granules of *China Rubra 5CH* three times a day, warding off bleeding, fever and fatigue.

To purify the liver and intestines, nothing beats the water that hospitals provide in abundance! Another source of unpleasant torment - as a woman — is when a catheter is inserted, with the possible irritation of the urethra. Just where pee comes out. Buy a tube of *Homeoplasmine*, intended for nasal burns. Apply it locally, as much as you want. I specify, not in the nasal mucosa! It's awesome! I asked the doctors, who gave their agreement because there are no side effects from it. By the way, this cream can be used during cystitis, when it burns after peeing.

Despite mandatory compression stockings in hospital, legs are sometimes painful. I take with me my *Lyman 50000* cream and it relieves me a lot. I continue using it throughout the year, having had a saphenous operation.

Personally, despite suffering from a postoperative iron deficiency, I preferred light meals to red meat. This is especially pertinent to those who, like me, have liver problems or never eat meat. The exception is, and this is true of everything: if you feel like having it and your body craves it. Or even your soul! There are many natural iron supplements, such as *Floradix* (natural). Recently I had a dose of *Maltofer*, (more full-bodied); both had no side effects. But if necessary, there is (I had it myself on another occasion) the drip, with just the iron in it. Obviously prescribed by your doctor!

Even without hepatic care, and with respect to your opinions, I'm not convinced that "eat all and anything" is a good path to take. The body will pay for it, whether you're healthy or not! Of course, here again, it is a subject that requires everyone to adapt the advice according to their own experience and feelings. Even if ... during hospital stays and post-operative shock, the feeling can be "a little distorted" ...

Being well prepared also includes experimenting beforehand with the two crutches that will accompany you. (About six weeks was the duration in 2002). I really advise you to exercise a little, because there is a proper way of moving. It consists of advancing one leg and the opposite crutch.

Another help, (for about £90), is a suitable cushion, which you can place anywhere when you sit down.

And above all, I recommend, (for about £60), a "grabber-stick". It will allow you to pick up what you dropped, because don't even think about lowering yourself right away.

Finally, if you have serious back problems, ask that a special mattress be placed on your bed, because you will inevitably have to stay (six weeks in 2002), without lying on your side.

Soon, it will be the physio ... walking ... and ... the cure!

Liberation! All those who have undergone this operation bear witness to this! What a delight to walk again ... freely!

So ... rejoice! It will be fast!

At the time of writing, it is exactly 15 years since I first walked with my prosthetic. It never annoys me. I passed the routine x-ray check-up after 15 years. Virtually nothing had moved and the surgeon told me to come back in five years.

There we go, I have now arrived at what carries us:

The Spine...and Spondylodesis (2009)

It is certain that, even if the back is operated on for a long time and each time is better and better, it will not be the same as the routine hip operation!

It is therefore important to take your time. To seek a surgeon who is renowned for the kind of operation you will undergo. Take documents with you, so as to ask relevant questions. My operation of November 2009 was, as already stated, inevitable.

A narrow canal, hernias, discs worn or non-existent. I moved again only with my crutches and often moaning with pain. Everything was tested in advance, including having injections under x-ray. These made it easier to locate all the different, damaged areas.

As for advice on anaesthesia, constipation, irritation of the urethra etc ... I refer you to the hip operation.

Of course, and once again, each case will be different. It is however beneficial that you learn about the details of the post-operative period. How many days of immobility? I would add that it is better to anticipate more rather than fewer days. It is best to be pleasantly surprised!

Then, especially if you don't have anyone close to you, dedicated to being with you almost constantly during your hospital stay, it is good to have the things that you'll need to hand. Accept that you will not be able to stand up or go forward, because it is fundamental that at the beginning, the "assembly" is welded well. In principle it is not a spa cure, but still buy a bottle of water spray and a good moisturizer. There will be a bell to ring by your bed for when you want something. Since I did not want to ring whenever my quilt needed adjusting, I tied one of the ends of it to a long, thin scarf, which allowed me to push back the quilt and pull it up with my scarf. I had also brought with me, and this helped me during the first nights, a small plastic ball, with "spades". Ping pong ball size. I think it's recommended for finger gymnastics. At night, I squeezed it to circulate my blood and ... move what I could move. Beneficial, too, are head massages. You can do them every day. And ... then ... as soon as possible, begin your breathing exercises.

When you are in rehabilitation, do not be discouraged! Do your physiotherapy with perseverance. Two pitfalls to avoid, when you exercise alone. Too much and too little. No excess. In general, there is a golden rule for physio: of course it's tiring, it's demanding and the muscles must be built up or rebuilt. But if it gets painful, never force yourself through it! And do not improvise anything! There are positions, attitudes to acquire, so as not to undo all the good. It's important, at least in the beginning, that what you are told to do is followed, and followed well.

As soon as you can do it, walking will be recommended. For a long time, the most delicate position will be the sitting position, while the standing and extended positions will be more suitable. A sloping cushion was an effective help for me, and today I still use it, when I'm sitting in the office or the car.

If you have the chance to have someone massage your feet ... Exquisite!

And above all, as soon as the dressing is removed from around your scar, it is heavenly to gently massage the area, so that the blood circulates! I remember the first gentle massage, around my incision, a real resurrection of the flesh!

However, do not put the scar in contact with water, before it is properly closed over. This mistake was made by a nurse for my hip and the scar remained blistered.

Patience, more than ever, and diligence! Also know, that we can be helped, if there has been a postoperative psychological shock ... Personally, I am always happy to leave the hospital only to find myself lost and worried, when I'm no longer there! I think it's a natural reaction. However, this operation does not require the same psychological approach as that of cancer. It is easy to understand. Especially since you will feel your body fortify each day ...

When your gown is off remember that, in fact, it never happened. It's a back that is not new, but repaired, which is now yours! It is high time that you give it your attention. Respecting the usual advice: wear a backpack, bend and sit properly, no sudden movements etc ... It is mandatory that you continue to walk and do your physio, as long as you can get up! This is really one of the first conditions for living with your new back again. For as long as possible! And, of course, it is imperative not to gain weight, thereby continually imposing loads. Imagine tying around six, seven, ten, twenty kilos of potatoes around your waist every day! Try it, put four on and go for a walk ...

Finally, especially if you are getting older, do some balance exercises, because over the years, one loses it and it is not the best time to fall. This is one of the easiest, and it only takes a few seconds a day: walk very small steps, one foot in front of the other, following a straight line. A line of your parquet flooring, or your kitchen tiles: in short in your apartment if possible, rather than on the highway ...

It seems logical that you don't run on tarmac, inflicting shocks on your replacement discs. Besides daily physiotherapy, walking and swimming seem to me the best sports. Swimming, if possible on your back, with light flippers.

I'm intentionally not listing my own daily physiotherapy exercises because there is a programme for each case. Simply, at the end of my programme, I have two or three exercises to rest and relax my back. Get in touch with your physiotherapist. The only exercise that I think I can share without any danger (but this must be verified for you), is a "universal" exercise. It will not only affect the health of your back, but also - especially if you are a woman – that of your bladder (preventing incontinence). This exercise can also improve your intestinal transit. It's about "carving" a natural lap belt, doing an exercise as often as you can, anywhere, whether you're sitting, standing or lying down. Of course, you're not going to begin by doing two hundred while you're finishing this book! The more you have fortified this natural lap belt, the more it will become second nature and you'll notice that you even perform your other exercises with it – the ones that are recommended! It's very simple: concentrate on your lower abdomen. Imagine that you need the toilet urgently, to empty your bladder as well as your intestines. There's aren't any recommended places for this, so then you will need to restrain yourself and fully contract the muscles of your lower abdomen counting to ten. Then a break, and you start again. You can, at first, put both hands on your lower abdomen, to feel the contractions. I insist, this "abdominal belt" woven from muscles, as deeply as possible, must become your basic support! The surgeon told me, during my last visit, that this deep bodybuilding even manages to reach the vertebrae. Also, the more you flex your thigh muscles, the easier it will be for you to get up with these, and not with your spine! And maybe, with this programme, you'll be able to get a job as a model! But ... beware of being discouraged, because with the years, you have to go a very "long way" to find the muscles!

Inquire, obey, and be aware. You walk now without suffering ... You know that the border is as thin as the line you follow on your parquet flooring, so put your best foot forward.

And then, know that there have been, are, and always will be rainy days! I can tell you that I went through more than one! You may have slept poorly, your morale might be right down in your boots or you will feel really fed up! On the one hand, you need to open your umbrella! Also allow yourself an "off" day. But from experience, whenever I was in this state of feeling my soul discouraged - I would get down on the carpet for my exercises, and my body won! Each time it was my body that strengthened my soul and reassured it. There is extraordinary interaction, but it is too often considered to be one way. Through the blessed lorgnette of tuppence ha'penny psychology! "If your morale goes, everything goes, so we can see that it's all in your head!"

"Well no, the body, especially so if you do exercises that are based on breathing, the body will boost your soul! Of course ... it's the body that remains the lynchpin ... and that will encourage you to not forget to live!

To re-live ...

Yes...

Relive!

Live ...

Kyphoplasty

After a broken vertebra, an operation is required as soon as possible! There is a waiting time that must not be exceeded. I had mine, six weeks after the fracture.

Gentle, compared to spondylodesis. But it still needs an anaesthetic. Even if two thousand imbeciles have gone through it before you with their fingers up their noses! Yes, of course I'm saying "imbeciles" without thinking. But you are still going to find people who will give you their opinion. Cousins and second cousins, a grandfather or great-grandmother who will have gone through it like flowers! While only those who have suffered, know what it is. Once again, each case is absolutely unique. A spine that has already been operated on will be more troublesome than a young spine on its first accident.

For me, it's more my entire spine, especially with the spondylodesis, but it's also the other cervical and lumbar weaknesses, which annoyed me the most!

Kyphoplasty was performed by my favourite champion, successfully. In addition, there were just two small holes on each side of the broken vertebra, so no big deal! I was able to move in my bed from the second day, as well as get up and leave the hospital four days later!

But ... there it is ... hello deception! I imagined myself taking back my life, as I was before the break! No chance! Three weeks of gentle walking, rest, pain while sitting, painkillers ...

And physio?

My dear physio ... well, I had to start again from zero!

Zero!

Even today, more than five months after the operation, I continue to "climb" the rungs of the ladder, patiently, one by one ...

The pain, however, has almost disappeared and the post-operative check, two months after the operation, is impeccable. It remains fragile and also a worry, and there are still muscular pains, which force me to rest or to change position. However, I live as I did before, with a little more fragility and more prudence. As the surgeon told me, with a back, I will always feel it!

That's why I insist, especially for congeners, that from a certain age we must do everything preventative that we can!

That being said, once again, long live science and long live surgery! In the old days, we would glue ourselves together the best we could, and the whole back would slip, until it became more and more curved!

So much for orthopedics ... Now I come to ...

Breast Cancer

You're not the first ... But ... what's the difference?

It's you ... you ... who's been hit ... So ...

So the battle is triggered!

Above all, I want to shout out some banal advice: prevention, prevention, prevention!

Long live screening, especially if you have a history. But also if you don't have one, which was my case!

I do not want to influence anybody, whether on

contraception or on how to manage the menopause. Personally, I was stuffed full with contraceptive pills between the ages of 20 and 30. I don't think I would do that anymore, even though they were the first pills of the '70s and research has advanced in this area as well. I remember that in the first month, my breasts were beautiful and inflated, doubled ... I found it sexy ... and did not complain!

Then, at age 45, four years after the removal of my womb, so as to be fitter and eternally young, I started hormone replacement therapy. Without doing any preliminary dosing. My cancer was hormone-dependent. Which doesn't mean that it wouldn't have ruptured ... but in any case, it was well fed!

So vigilance! Inquire about natural "oestrogens" too, especially in dietary supplements of soy, the isoflavones. Know that scientific advice is divided. Additionally, they are not recommended if you have had a breast tumour.

As for breast cancer, there are so many, I could almost say one for each of us! Therefore, it would be absolutely pointless to give any advice whatsoever, on the operating methods or the medical treatments. Anyway, reserve that for specialists! I must still clarify that I escaped the mastectomy due to split opinions.

But once again, each case is unique, wherever you are! Yes, wherever you are! Fortunately! I remember the great surgeon, the best, who said to me: "We now have a global protocol and scientists are exchanging ideas continuously in discussions."

So trust: but this doesn't prevent you from seeking a second opinion ...

I must add, to be honest, that I mobilised all my contacts in the medical community, but also ... my "links with the invisible"! Orthodox Christian, I immediately asked all my friends to pray for me. And I prayed too, for my doctors ...

Whatever your beliefs, you will dive into this unknown ... Anyway, you have no choice! But you are lucky enough to be in a country, where you are cared for, healed and kept company ...

The operation is behind you?

Bravo! Now you breathe and you continue the fight!

I can, alas, only enlighten you a little, once again, with my experience.

If you undergoing x-rays, don't worry! Everything will be fine.

At worst, there will be a big sunburn on the breast. You will be told what to apply. I escaped chemo, even though the opinions were not unanimous. Today, 16 years later, I am happy with the choice. So I will limit myself to mentioning some tips about the treatments that I received. Apart from that ... during the summer of 2016, I accompanied my dear brother, for two chemos, the most powerful that exist, against acute leukaemia. Once again, there are no comparisons and everyone is different. In addition, he displayed extraordinary humour and courage. But I must say that the word terrifies ... and it is ... terrifying ... but not insurmountable! Especially since there are less aggressive chemos for many breast cancers.

On the other hand, I benefited from seven and a half years of treatment.

First was two and a half years of *Tamoxifen*, followed by five years of *Arimidex*.

The beginning was difficult. Under replacement hormones, the racing car was launched in the opposite direction. Hello menopause TGV! With its panoply of small delights that occur very quickly ... But again, each will react in their own way. The body has an incredible ability to bounce back ... The spirit too ... even though it must be piloted sometimes. I read and quickly threw in the trash, then forgot, the miseries that could occur, as indicated on the leaflet! Ditto for the *Arimidex* ... Also, apart from the fact that it was not the makeover of my life, I can only thank science, once again, for these treatments that are used on thousands of women ...

I urge you to carefully write a personal health record. The doctors will thank you. You will collaborate to the maximum. On this passport, besides your name, your insurance, your weight, your height and your blood type, your next of kin, write down everything that you have had since childhood. Including serious treatments or surgeries. This will be a valuable source of information.

Good, you can also do like an old English friend of my parents in Kenya:

Doctor: "So, Madam, what brings you here? "

"Well, you idiot, it's up to you to tell me!"

Personally, I update my card, whenever it is necessary, and I always carry a miniature copy of it on me!

In my research, I first came upon the famous book by Dr. David Servan-Schreiber, *Anticancer*, and so its many tips and recipes are part of my daily life. This rich book is a living testimony and has a special place in my library, although I will mention others, more recent and complementary. In addition, he had a terrifying cancer (a brain tumor). He lived on for about 22 years, though his prognosis had only allowed him six months! And then, he was patient, doctor and scientist. Sometimes, some passages are too scientific, but it is worth reading. Furthermore his diet, as already mentioned above, will promote a good cardiovascular system and provide good support against osteoarthritis. However, it is essential to discuss this with your oncologist and your doctor. And to inform them of important changes that are made.

In his book, Dr. Servan-Schreiber insists on some facts that have since become famous, namely: ban refined sugars and flours, light products, popcorn (GMOs). Limit cow's milk, salt, gluten, red meats, hydrogenated oils and margarines. Limit animal fat. (American researchers recently talked about reducing them to 20% of total calories.) And ... of course, this crap tobacco! When we are a bit too lazy to prepare our meals or peel our fruits, we must be careful with the salt and sugars hidden in the industrial fruit juices, cornflakes, mueslis, the famous energy bars and all "ready meals", even organic ones.

The food and advice that I will enumerate, are taken from his book, but also from the two books that I will also present briefly. Here and there, I will mention other authors, because books on health are not lacking.

The second book is that by Professor David Khayat: *The Real Anticancer Regime*. We sometimes oppose the two books, in my opinion wrongly! It is a very scientific book in some respects (cancer development etc ...) and I sometimes had trouble following it. But there are clear and targeted prevention tips. For example, on page 17 of its introduction: "Because the truth is there: our eating habits, taken in a broad sense, are actually responsible for many of the cancers we develop". At the same time, it remains antithetical, an attitude that suits me perfectly. Thus in his conclusion, page 261, he declares: "I do not agree with this attitude, this posture which consists of being afraid of everything, of being ready to give up everything, provided that we are very calm in our life!" I will often return to this antinomy between the fight to prevent (including recurrence), the change of life and habits, and at the same time not forgetting to live! It sounds banal, but it's not easy at all! The very accessible part of his book is about nutrition tips, food charts, easy to remember. Professor Khayat is still practising and ... for the human interest story, he was Johnny Halliday's last doctor!

I have consulted several other books, and here it is up to everyone to expand their research. We will see that we finish little, always coming back to the same recommendations. But I still want to quote a book that was precious to me, that of the doctors Richard Béliveau and Denis Gingras: *The Anti-Cancer Method*. For me, the book is the most accessible and easy to put into practice. This book is not only for those who are suffering from cancer, but also for those who want to become aware of the importance of prevention in our civilised world! "We all have tumours" (page 17) ... but ... "To reach a mature stage, a cancer must be able to count on the collaboration of its environment ..." (page 23). I will immediately enumerate the ten golden rules found in this book for establishing informed prevention:

- Do not smoke.
- Have a body mass index of between 21 and 23.

- Do not consume more than 500g of red meat a week.[5]
- Eat plenty of fruit and vegetables.
- Have at least 30 minutes of physical activity a day.
- Do not drink more than two glasses of alcohol per day, one for women, and preferably wine.
- Limit products preserved in salt.
- Have sufficient preventive sun protection.
- In place of all-round food supplements, a healthy and varied diet.
- Follow these tips to the letter to avoid recurrence.

I will not summarise these good books, which everyone can buy and read. You can even listen to excerpts from conferences on *YouTube*. On the other hand, I will list a number of drinks and foods that are recommended. Of course, I mostly remembered those related to breast cancer. But we can expand the range, without really being wrong. For example, flaxseed, pomegranate and concentrated tomato sauce are also three dietary precautions against prostate cancer.

I try to consume every day, in small quantities, a dozen of these foods and drinks. I eat them raw, or lightly cooked (gently steamed). I also take some food supplements. Pomegranate capsules, because the juice is quite rare. My iron rate is often very low. So I take supplements, but apart from when I have a deficiency, I take them naturally. (Genus *Floradix* or, more recently, homeopathic preparations.) Vitamin D3, 12 drops every day, and that is with the agreement of my oncologist. A magnesium tablet in the evening. And osteoporosis requires 1000 mg of calcium a day. 500 mg in the morning, 500 mg in the evening. With regard to dietary supplements, opinions are controversial. Professor Khayat recommends them, for one simple reason: it would be necessary to consume impracticably large quantities of these anti-cancer foods for them to be therapeutic. Dr. Béliveau and Dr. Gingras prefer daily food, which is a form of long-term prevention. My two doctors from

---

[5] Be careful with age to control your intake and eventual lack of vitamin B12, present in animal fats.

Bordeaux, a homeopath and an internist, recommended them. For another obvious reason too, modern food is so stripped of its properties. Once again, it depends on the age, the possibilities and specificities of each one and it is advisable to speak with a specialist.

Although I try to follow this diet with great regularity, once a week, I eat whatever I like! Without going mad though, with a ton of ice cream or chips with mayonnaise!

Before listing, we can add that we must avoid pickled foods, smoked, fried, prepared dishes, woks, barbecues and pesticides. Smoking! The cigarette is carcinogenic, from the first puff! My God, if you have not started, never begin. Know this too, it will screw up your mouth, and enslave you. Because there are addictive substances in cigarettes! "By manipulating tobacco to increase its addictive properties, the tobacco industry has created what is possibly the most devastating weapon in the history of mankind."[6] Also take care with water that has stagnated in plastic bottles in the heat or even with the tap water in some areas.

Finally, I have limited myself on principal to "the most valiant soldiers"!

The best fruits for breast cancer are peaches and small berries (strawberries, blueberries, blackberries, raspberries, cranberries). They can be frozen or even made into jams. Pomegranate juice or dietary supplements. Mangos and citrus fruits.

The flagship vegetable: broccoli! Bad luck, personally it's the only vegetable I hate! So I find it, either powdered for making soup or for mixing with juice (organic), or I sprout seeds and eat a tablespoon a day. Its effectiveness would be enhanced if you eat tomato sauce at the same meal. But all the other crucifers are also very good soldiers.

Soy, if you have already had breast cancer, but it should not be abused and in this case, especially not in supplement form as isoflavones. I read that it should not be taken during chemo. On

---

[6] Dr. Richard Béliveau and Denis Gingras, *La méthode anticancer*, page 46

the other hand, mushrooms and algae intensify its effect.

Seeds, and the essentials are flaxseed. But beware, they deteriorate quickly. They must be kept in the fridge. I grind two teaspoons each morning. I eat them with some soy and other recommended seeds, like squash, sunflower, sesame, chia seeds.

The flagship anti-cancer drink: green tea! But, for it to keep its properties, do not pour it into boiling water. The water should be around 60°c. Green tea (preferably Japanese), should also enhance the effectiveness of x-rays. But take care with calcium absorption. Better to drink it two hours before or after taking calcium. Its effectiveness would be further increased with lemon, which is another potent anticancer food. Remember, however, that lemon juice likes to eat a lot of tooth enamel! It's also recommended to drink green tea and, at the same meal, consume soy. The coffee looks great too, but again, watch out for calcium absorption.

Algae, for those who can bear them. At home, they go well when they are dried and I can sprinkle them on my salads or Miso soup (fermented soy soup). Yes, Miso, I take it in the form of soup and that makes me feel good when I have intestinal bloating or a little nausea. But it is imperative to take real Miso: in general, only health food shops sell it!

Resveratrol, found in red wine (no more than one drink a day). As I don't drink any more, since hepatitis C, I drink some organic grape juice, or take resveratrol in peanuts, blackberries, cranberries, black grapes and raspberries.

The key spices: turmeric and ginger. It is imperative to consume turmeric with black pepper and in olive oil. Its effectiveness is at least a thousand times more powerful. As for ginger, I cut it into small pieces and boil it for about three minutes. You can add lemon, cinnamon or even green tea to this drink.

For the "sweet-toothed": four squares per day of dark chocolate, minimum 70% cocoa.

Cinnamon too, is an excellent anti-cancer spice. It complements soy yogurts and plain tofu. But also apple sauce, herbal teas, tea. Use Ceylon cinnamon, organic if possible.

Mushrooms are good fighters, especially oyster mushrooms for breast cancer.

Spices, such as thyme (in addition to being stuffed full with calcium), paprika, rosemary.

Omega 3 with fish, sardines, organic salmon, mackerel. A quick anti-cancer recipe: I mix canned sardines with sweet potatoes, turmeric, pepper and olive oil.

Almonds, hazelnuts and especially nuts. Brazil nuts contain a lot of selenium that increases the effect of chemo and is an excellent anti-cancer food in itself

I already mentioned vitamin D3. Especially if you've had breast cancer. Even more so, if you don't regularly take the sun!

For all cancers, you can add garlic. Personally, I digest it very badly. If you can tolerate it, it is recommended to crush a clove with a fork. Let it macerate for ten minutes in its juice, (the anti-cancer molecules are then released). Then mix with olive oil. Yes, olive oil: a must-have soldier too!

Legumes: lentils, chickpeas, beans etc.

Onions, leeks, watercress, cucumber, radish, squash and once again all species of cabbage, with broccoli in the lead! "Chinese women who consume more crucifers see their risk of developing breast cancer halved..."[7]

It is important to combine and especially to diversify foods.

Drink enough water, of course. The ideal would be to start the day with a large glass and finish with a drink, before bedtime.

I also drink herbal teas: sage, nettle, mint.

Of course, just because a food is healthy does not mean that you have to abuse it.

Try to be measured. Ask your doctor and ... have fun too!

Another soldier - or better still, a colonel - who doesn't relate to food is unanimously accepted: movement! Cancer loves tranquility! We recommend a minimum of 2.5 hours of

---

[7] Doctors Gingras and Béliveau, *Les aliments contre le cancer*, page 83

sustained activity per week. In fact, if you walk at an accelerated pace, every day for 30 minutes the tour has already been played!

Some doctors — see, amongst that of others, the research of "City of Hope" in Los Angeles - advise taking about 240 mg, 3x81mg, of aspirin a week. Especially so when tumours are active, or to reduce the risk of a recurrence of hormonal breast cancer. What's more, from a certain age it will have a beneficial effect on blood flow. It is necessary to discuss this possible route with a doctor.

And ... the Mind ...

It has been scientifically proven (see, among others, David Servan-Schreiber's book), that volunteers reciting daily Tibetan mantras or other repetitive prayers have a much better heart rate and a stronger immune system! Because to fight against cancer, it is obvious that it is worth fighting against other diseases. Including all forms of inflammation!

In practical terms, I want to mention educating the mind in the taking on of certain priorities. The renouncing of many material advantages. To the profit of the best health insurance (in Switzerland it's private, so exorbitantly priced!), certified quality food, food supplements and alternative treatments are not reimbursed, neither is an orthopaedic bed etc....

I will come back to the central theme of the mind, but it is obligatory to take the following into account. This is the only complaint I would make to the fabulous team, so humane, who supported my dear brother. They did not insist enough on psychological support. He didn't trust it because his suffering was so deep and established ...

Again, drawing conclusions about illness or recurrence ... or ... even healing seems monstrous to me. Especially coming from brave fools who do not know what that represents. But, as a patient, neglecting the emotional side, the psychological side (without capsizing in your own navel), even the spiritual side, is really to fall back into confinement. And to cut oneself off from sources of energy, support, joy ... and eventual healing.

A few words on:

Hepatitis C

Quickly, because I was lucky enough to be one of those in whom it "healed spontaneously". Which of course, means that I did not have to be vigilant, or follow a suitable diet.

It seems to be only the chronic viral disease that can be cured with antivirals. It should be known, however, that this disease can lead to cirrhosis of the liver and/or cancer. So, we are not kidding! Not to scare you, but so that you can understand that the first recommendation of my doctor, namely, not to consume alcohol, especially as a woman, was an immediate decision. I have not touched a drop of alcohol for 20 years! The good news is that the anti-cancer, anti-osteoarthritis diet is also a good strategy for the liver! You spare it grills, carbonnades, animal fats, fried foods, dangerous edible oils and all the bad sugars. You give it fresh fruit and vegetables, water and it is satisfied!

As a natural remedy, *phosphorus 15 CH*, of which I regularly take a four-week course, one dose (or ten granules) each week.

I constantly take before breakfast and lunch, capsules of either milk thistle or artichoke. Also, in the spring, I take doses of black radish. (Drinking a lot because it is diuretic.) Two or three tablets of spirulina daily, quickly swallowed, because its smell repulses me, its taste too. But it seems to be a precious seaweed, not just for the liver. What works well for me twice a year, is a three-week course of *Desmodium*: 5 ml in the morning in a glass of warm water and 5 ml in the evening. Obviously, again, you have to drink a lot of water and not combine the treatment with bountiful meals. When I take mine, I am on a light diet, based on many sweet steamed vegetables, especially leeks, endives, broccoli, sweet potatoes, dandelions, fennel, spinach. But also raves, carrots and raw red beets, grated. As well as fruits, mangos, avocados, bananas ... and always apples!

Garlic, if you can bear it. I also take *Desmodium*, after strong drugs or anaesthesia.

For "biliary emptying", since my childhood … I have placed a hot water bottle over my liver, ten minutes before falling asleep. It's something I got from my dear mum!

I add, since I am going to speak also of the psychic, that all that damages your heart, will also damage your liver. We can't change our sensitivity, I'm sure of that, but we must try to manage it accordingly … More easily written than done!

I still wish, since we are talking about health, to share a heap of advice that I practice permanently for other ills. Once again, nothing exhaustive and everyone must check it and enrich it! At the slightest doubt, consult the advice of your doctor rather than improvise!

Bronchitis, Asthma, Pneumonia and Respiratory Infections

Not funny! Especially, when the years get involved!

If you smoke, you know the dangers …

Do everything you can and more, to do without this scourge.

I come back again to breathing: whatever the method, take daily breaths.

But it is important, if you suffer from asthma or bronchitis, to learn to breathe with the upper part of your chest. And no, only abdominal breathing. These breathing exercises must become a routine.

Concerning asthma, you can have blood tests to detect possible allergies.

If you have the chance of swimming in an almost clean sea, do not hesitate to dive in, to fill your nostrils once or twice during each swim and then fly!

Sage tea, excellent for many things, can be one of your daily herbal teas.

The famous course of *Desmodium* for the liver (5ml in the morning and 5ml in the evening in a glass of water), is also beneficial for the bronchi.

And that of thyme with lemon juice, at the first warning.

Equally, turmeric with a little honey. A teaspoon every hour at the beginning, then space it out. Before swallowing, let it melt in your mouth. But you should know that turmeric can cause heartburn and also acts as an anticoagulant. So ask the doctor if you are being treated with anticoagulants. Anyway, I repeat the need to be measured in everything ... and check, check, check ...

Don't feel embarrassed, during epidemics, about wearing a mask in those places that are at risk!

Asians, in many countries, don't part company with them!

Without becoming obsessed with the white tornado, wash and disinfect your hands as soon as you touch surfaces at risk, that is to say, everything in times of contagion.

For two or three pounds one can buy mini bottles of hand sanitiser everywhere. I do not deprive myself of this!

As a preventative, to strengthen me, from November to March I take yeast, *Strath* (two tablets before breakfast and two before lunch) and Vitamin C *Acerola*. But if illness is apparent, I take 1000 mg of synthetic vitamin C twice in fresh orange juice. (Recipe from my homeopath in Bordeaux).

There is of course for the followers, homeopathic vaccines. I used them a long time but for the past two years (in consideration of my age and my fragility) I get vaccinated: a) against flu, every year and b) against pneumonia, every five years. I have stopped this, but I also did a three-month course of *Broncho-Vaxom*, one tablet for ten days each winter month.

I always have on me, summer and winter, a few tablets, like Strepsil, to disinfect me, at the slightest sign of a throat that scratches! And I wear a scarf all year, night and day, to avoid throat chills.

Do not forget that a train or air-conditioned public transport in the middle of the summer is as dangerous or more dangerous than the first cold.

Almost the whole year round, I rub the soles of my feet with Vicks' *Vaporub*, before sleeping.

With essential oils, I rub my wrist in winter with *Ravintsara*. Often I use a diffuser with eucalyptus and thyme. Thyme, I try to drink it all the winter. Especially since it contains a lot of plant calcium.

From the first warning signs, we should stop dairy products as they promote inflammation. It seems that mother tincture of bramble helps. Also grated black radish, macerated at night in honey so as to drink the juice in the morning. I have not tried this because for me, with my history and asthma, the first alert means immediate recourse to my cortisone spray, or even antibiotics, if my doctor deems it necessary. I'm relieved when I do not have to add oral cortisone!

As already stated, all infections and inflammations are to be taken very seriously, especially when you have had cancer.

So much for the bronchi.

A Word about the Colon

It is essential, especially if you have health concerns, not to be constipated! Pelvic floor exercises will help you. I also advise you to try to empty your colon at regular intervals. In the morning after breakfast, for example. On an empty stomach, while standing up, a large glass of warm water can contribute to this. I take very long treatments, nettle tea fasting. I add a little lemon juice[8] and drink it lukewarm. Three times a year, I drink a dose of aloe mixed with fig juice on an empty stomach for three weeks. If constipation is watching me, especially while traveling, then I use a glycerine suppository. Sometimes I soak dried prunes and figs at night. I eat them in the morning, before breakfast. Ground flaxseeds in the morning help a lot. And then I learned how to empty my colon with the books of Dr. Frédéric Saldmann, (very practical books). We must get back to how things were "before the modern toilets". Squatting, as in

---

[8] After the lemon juice, rinse your mouth, without washing your teeth immediately, to avoid damaging the tooth enamel.

Turkish toilets. To get into this position, without transforming the toilet, just place a small stool under your feet.

Avocado is an excellent food and balm for the intestines. It can replace butter or mayonnaise, as a sandwich base.

Above all, I hydrate myself with the famous litre and a half of water every day! This regular hydration also allows me to reduce the risks of:

Cystitis

With age, this often becomes a disabling worry.

Some really basic tips: impeccable hygiene, without killing the flora of the necessary bacteria. Beware of heat and sweating. Also avoid cold and icy floors. I was a fan of the electric cushion, but I gave up because I slept with it, which is not recommended. However, during alerts, I put a hot water bottle on my lower abdomen. I bought a "baby hot water bottle model" and I slip it into my suitcase when I travel. Although the benefits have recently been controversial, I do a course of cranberry juice (either in the form of tablets or, better, dried berries) at the slightest suspicion of it. I also consume more cinnamon than usual, which would seem to have a mild and natural antibiotic effect.

Also at the slightest warning, I apply a little *Homeoplasmine* (as I indicated after the positioning of a probe). Sometimes, I even apply it preventively. It is also important to take your time (especially at night, if you are half asleep on your toilet bowl!), to empty the bladder. Even if you have to wait and start over again. At the same time, one can do an exercise that will strengthen the muscle tone, to avoid urinary incontinence. Very easy: in the middle of a jet, you instantly stop urination and count to ten. Then you continue to urinate normally.

Another exercise to strengthen your perineum: several times a day, sitting in your car or elsewhere, you contract the muscles of your lower abdomen, as if to restrain yourself from going to the bathroom. You count to ten and rest. (Exercise indicated above for your spine).

Finally, there are now tests that you can do alone, to detect infections that should direct you to see a doctor.

Circulation: especially, that of the legs

All the doctors to whom I put the question about *class 2 compression stockings*, since the two saphenous veins were removed and about forty varicose veins at the age of 46, are unanimous: what is better!

I have worn them for twenty years! Compression stockings (up to the top of the thigh) for the summer and tights (always compression 2, qualified medical and reimbursed by health insurance), for the winter. I cannot do without them! This avoids swollen and painful legs, and so far (for 21 years), no relapse. But still we must hang on! This is not an obvious discipline, even if it becomes a habit. Especially at first, you have to find the right way of putting them on. Me, I lay down a few minutes after the shower, then equipped with rubber gloves, I put them in positions that are not at all erotic ... The material neither, even if there was to be huge progress in the field. Frankly, the stockings or pantyhose on the current market are confused with leggings or opaque tights! I would say, they refine (and for good reason), the shape of your pins! Natural remedy and more!

Pay attention, if you are going to be operated on and limited in your movements (back, hip). I bought some kind of "sock-horn" and I always practice with it before the operation.

In the natural field there is, if you can bear it, the alternating hot-cold showers. In summer, I always try to end my shower with a good cold jet on my legs. Several times a day, and especially if I've been sitting, I get up, barefooted or with warm slippers and I go back and forth on tiptoe, while standing against the back of the chair. And of course: to move ... to walk ... to swim ... to ride a bike or, as my dear mother did at 87, pedalling in bed, legs in the air. If your back allows it, press your legs down on the wall and rest for a few minutes.

As medicine for circulation, I take *Daflon 500*, alternating with horse chestnut, and *Pygenol*. There are plenty of them, chemical or natural. But it seems that we must change between them regularly, for them to bring the best possible improvement.

As for foods, we must focus on those rich in vitamin E, such as nuts. It seems that turmeric is also a natural anticoagulant, as I said before.

In the evening, I never fail to moisturise my legs, massaging them a little. Either with a plain moisturising cream, or with a cream or a gel for the circulation of the blood (in summer the gel is fresh but it dries). When traveling by plane, I get up, at least once every hour and walk down the gangway. In the car, I take a few steps every two, three hours. If a very long flight is planned, you can talk to your doctor, who may give you an injection to thin the blood (*Heparin* or something else). The sort we have when we are operated on and remain motionless.

And if you have the chance now and again of a course of reflexology, it's great. Besides, it's not just for the legs and circulation! But it is essential to find the rare pearl ... more and more rare! Otherwise, look for a good soul, with good hands that will massage you a little, regularly, on your feet and legs.

I'm taking this opportunity for an aside. Whenever your body gets hurt, (because we are not talking here about bodies in top form!), if it is massaged, touched, caressed, it will be a balm and a resurrection. A dull example, my hands and my wrists, full of osteoarthritis, become more and more painful. So when I can, I cover them with olive oil, and massage them for about ten minutes.

You're going to tell me rightly, that all this is eating up time and that the days are going by. Yes, it's true, but there are so many minutes that we waste in a day ... not doing well, even doing harm. I will come back to it later, but that's for you to care about, on your side of the fence! It's a bit like that, this complicit enemy! Realise - and it often happens only during the shock of an illness - that you *can* tame your body and help it to fight actively.

I still wish to add to this a few pieces of advice or help that I practice regularly.

During operations or serious illnesses (which for me start with a good bout of bronchitis), the liver and also the stomach are affected.

For the stomach, apart from those difficult times, where only the famous proton pumps are effective, I became familiar with *Gaviscon*, which is nothing but sodium bicarbonate tablets. But in homeopathic doses. And it works! During stomach disorders, night awakenings, following gastric burns, I suck a quarter of a tablet and really, I am relieved. In case of heartburn, a tablespoon of sheep or goats' yogurt is also effective. A chicken broth can also soothe. And of course, a meal in the evening that does not include alcohol, pastries or fries. If possible, three hours before going to bed. I also try to respect the acid-base balance during meals. Basically, do not eat cereals or proteins alone, but combine them with a salad, vegetable or fruit. And then ... the golden rule, with which my adorable grandfather broke my ears: chew, chew, chew ...

To help with sleep, I often drink orange blossom tea, or suck valerian pastilles. I pour a few drops of lavender oil on my pillow.

We cannot repeat it enough: avoid bitterness, stress, resentment and gloomy thoughts. This is also true - although it is not the only remedy, especially if there are problems of congenital origin - for arrhythmia and tachycardia.

As side effects of some medications, or simply even long winters locked in an overheated room, one can end up with extremely dry eyes. With - I'm not kidding, it's the threat my ophthalmologist used if I didn't show myself to be diligently following my treatment - little holes in the eyes. Before this happens, you must be attentive and consult with a professional. There are many fantastic drops that can be applied - once again, with discipline - throughout the day. In the evening, an extraordinary vitamin A cream helps, with which eyes are painted before sleeping. I cannot live without it, despite the slimy look that it gives me!

And then something from my dear grandmother: small circular massages, all around the orbit, with the middle finger. We finish the massage by rubbing the two palms of the hands and placing them, heated, on the eyes.

To finish with the body, it is obvious that if you cross diseases, operations and ... old age, (as a friend of my dad's said: "The one who has nothing has only to wait!"), you will feel great blows of fatigue. I'm talking about physical fatigue right now. Knowing that certain deficits in vitamins and/or minerals, can also trigger psychological disorders. Also I advise making an assessment of iron levels, especially if you have been operated on. Depending on your diet, with more or less red meat, you can supplement with natural iron[9], such as *Floradix* for example. And if the exhaustion persists, why not a course of fortifiers? My favourite is *Strath*, with *Acerola* and magnesium for relaxation. To strengthen my immune system, echinacea treatment in winter. But, all that is no substitute for a life of good food and hygiene! Finally, I always take these food supplements with the consent of my doctor.

Before leaving the somatic, I would like to add something about:

The Brain

I do not pretend to know either its operation, or its universe! I simply advise everyone to learn about the prodigious discoveries of recent years. As I am going to talk about various activities, I would like to encourage any stimulation of the brain. At any age too! In the past, it was believed that, after fifty years, the neurons followed their wretched destiny of degeneration,

---

[9] Look to control the balance of other vitamins and minerals, above all in old age. (Vitamin B12, vitamin D, potassium, sodium, selenium, calcium, magnesium etc...)

without being remedied. I prefer to cite doctors. In a book very accessible to the general public, Anne Le Marchand, *Pamper your Brain*, writes: "Genes do not determine the fate of our brain. Throughout life, neuroplasticity allows our lifestyle and actions to play a central role in how the brain physically evolves." (Page 23). She speaks not only of hygiene, (food, respiratory, physical activity), but also of the heavy load of our repressed emotions, of chronic stress. Elements of which I will return to. But also the perils of isolation: "The development of the human brain feeds on social relationships" (Page 88). Beware of routine, dare to venture into the unknown, into the unexpected. Cultivate a liking for effort! In his book *Your Health Without Risk*, Dr. Frédéric Saldmann reports: "... Finnish scientists have shown that by supporting daily physical exercise, we made new neurons every day. (Page 185). Or again: "It is not by resting, that we will win neurons, but the opposite." (Page 196) As my dear brother said: "I want to grow old, but not by drawing sunflowers in an old people's home!" So, get started in any creative activity that suits your desires, before you get to the sunflowers! "Art and the process of creation, whether artistic or scientific, leads to and develops what is called psychological flexibility ... allowing us to face the difficulties inherent in life with a flexibility."[10] Everyone has gifts to develop. Even if ... it's not always obvious how to be inspired! Another adventure to try! I will add, if the reader has not already worked it out, that I chose, a few years ago, to reconnect with my youthful passion for writing ...

Before talking a little about my experiences with this other beautiful brain that is the Heart, I want to emphasise again, some practical elements of daily hygiene. Without becoming obsessed with viruses and bacteria!

Hygiene: an ally not to be despised

Paradoxically, if I think back to the time of my childhood and

10 Anne Le Marchand *Chouchoutez Votre Cerveau*, page 84.

the advice of my grandparents, it seems to me that our hygiene has not made any progress! Few children wash their hands before eating. Tablecloths that have disappeared from many restaurants, or these public places, which have taken on gigantic dimensions. They are so many meeting places for microbes and international bacteria! So a rule of thumb: I always have a small bottle of disinfectant on me and sanitise my hands several times a day. Especially while travelling.

If there isn't even a paper tablecloth on the restaurant table, I try to wipe it before putting down my cutlery. I am also careful with the glasses, or cups, from which I drink. I avoid sitting on any public toilets! Same caution in the plane! Especially with the low-cost airlines, which have only a few minutes to clean the cabin, before receiving the next passengers. Abroad, I always drink closed bottled water or boil it for at least five minutes. Having had, as I have already mentioned, a big issue once with water, I don't have the slightest doubt about also being careful with the water I use to brush my teeth. Even when showering, I let a little water flow before getting in.

I regularly disinfect my small medicine boxes.

However, I do not stay locked in at home. I will repeat again: prevention, caution, (especially if the immune system is fragile), but these things must not kill life ... which ... in any case will always be a risk ... and ... a permanent miracle!

At home, it is also possible to improve daily hygiene. When did you last clean your fridge? Recently, I clean it thoroughly every two months. Every week, I wipe a cloth with an alcohol-based disinfectant. In the same way, you have to think of cleaning your microwave regularly. But beware of sponges, nests *par excellence* for microbes and bacteria. Disinfect them, change them regularly or better, use household paper (recycled for ecology). Also take care of wet wipes, filled with bacteria, and towels.

As for fruit and vegetables, I peel them, if they are not organic. At the very least I rinse them for a few minutes in vinegar.

Body hygiene seems self-evident. In fact, we often paint ourselves with scented foams and we forget about the navel full of germs, the spaces between the toes and nostrils. We change perfumes, but we let the same toothbrush hang around for months, if possible close to the toilet bowl[11]. We brush our teeth quickly, one eye on our laptop and we neglect to floss, essential for good oral hygiene. Treated with bisphosphonates against osteoporosis, I am very attentive to the health of my mouth. Indeed, especially if one has suffered from cancer, it is recommended not to have a tooth extraction while under biphosphonates. I also try to brush my gums and tongue gently. Yes, I know, it takes a little time, but a trip to the dentist does too!

Finally, every week, I disinfect my cell phone and clean my glasses thoroughly.

This programme does not seem excessive to me. But it is obvious, that one can also wash and protect oneself too much. Even killing the flora and bacteria that are vital to our body! So be measured and use discernment.

I already said, during outbreaks of flu or other illnesses, I do not hesitate to wear a mask.

I insist once again on the most basic hygiene: that of life: breathing! Yes, if one day I don't do my deep breathing exercises, for only ten minutes, I feel that a part of my life has remained buried! I emphasise it again forcefully: be measured in everything! Do everything in moderation ... Learn to know your rhythms, the rhythms of the body ... and of the soul. In this regard, I convey the advice given to me by my oncologist: without obsession but consciously, observe the reactions of your body, changes, disorders. And when you suspect something's wrong it is better to consult about treatment. Once again: collaborate ...

I still want to incorporate mental hygiene into this paragraph about hygiene. The great danger of disabling illness, whatever it may be, is isolation. A dear friend, always beautifully turned out,

---

[11] Some of these points are taken from the books by Doctor Frédéric Saldmann, already referenced.

refuses since her illness to meet her friends, so that they don't see her in that state. And now this state has lasted for two years ... I understand this reaction, but apart from the fact that tranquillity is a major component of recovery, we must remember that any encounter with others is a grace.

A grace ...

Have the courage to move about, when you are moping. Even if you're able to handle loneliness. I would say, especially so! Because of course it is an asset, as long as it does not lead to withdrawal and the dangers of confinement. Go to others! In general, the crowd doesn't rush to be in front of the "degraded". This also applies to old age, which regardless of our state of health, is a humiliation. I remember my mother's words, always realistic and sometimes very raw. At that time, with an attractive physique and, through my profession, in contact with the big directors of banks and big firms, I was much courted.

"You'll see," Mum said to me, "when you're no longer eating at the big boys' table, in the same way that your friends will not find you that great!" And she was right! To take it down a notch, and be even more trivial, at 20 years of age all the males were jostling to carry my bags, without me even asking! See you soon, 70, "sort yourself out, old woman!" And yet, I often try to ... meet ... to enter into communion, while defining my timings! Because it's the only way to stay alive! Of course, everyone has their own rhythm ... and freedom! There are still flourishing recluses today ... There are also periods in our lives life, where we need to take stock alone and serenely. But beware, if the duration goes on too long ... As for morale, so important for the fight against diseases, it must remove itself from any form of depression. And if it clings to it, then ask for help.

Whatever your past genius, your admirers, you must have the courage to break out of your sense of pride, to ask for help. Not necessarily from those who are forcing you to reintegrate with their two-bit psychology. But search, just as for the body ... search, strike, go, scream! And ... I insist, declare war on your damn pride! And then ... entertain humour, whatever happens!

Whistle, sing, even if your voice sounds like a saucepan. Sing or whistle at least once a day. Whatever!

Finally, I recall once again, in this form of hygiene, the energy gained during creative activities. Not only do they divert thoughts related to illness, but they vivify and lead to all forms of communion.

Now I come to talk about the soul and ...

The Heart!

Although having completed a long analysis, followed courses in psychology and passed a bachelor's degree in theology, I am neither an expert nor a professional! All that I describe below comes again from my experience and ... from my daily conquests.

Trials, every suffering hurts...sometimes violently!

Again, everyone must determine this for themselves! My generation has often grown up with a scornful smile toward the sufferings of the soul. Psychotherapy was for the crazy! Religion for the illiterate and frustrated bigots! And ... above all, no antidepressants! While in a state of shock, or a difficult treatment, they can be a relief. In practically all hospitals now, counselling is on offer. Why not try it?

If we return to cancer, but also to any other big disease, or test in the broadest sense, at least it has now afforded you the right to open doors. Don't hold fast to your past "prisons". Maybe you must also start by accepting your weakness? "Resilience has nothing to do with invulnerability"[12]. And "exploit" this vulnerability, giving it the freedom to approach unexplored horizons! It is often said that stress is one of the factors favouring cancer. It is obvious that these deep angsts, which have marked our children's sufferings, are not a refuge of health! We can also decide to confront them. To finally give them the floor. And if they, in turn, become kinds of

[12] Boris Cyrulnik, *Un Merveilleux Malheur*, page 68.

accomplices? In transfiguring this darkened dirt, lurking in us. In his fascinating book *A Wonderful Misfortune*, Boris Cyrulnik, gives examples of children who, having lived the worst horrors, have rebounded. However, it does not limit this rebound to chance, be it genetic or otherwise! But to the meeting of a salvation figure, at a moment in their lives. It is still necessary to accept, to seize the outstretched hand! Leaving aside the pride of our own genius! Yes, yes, I persist in believing that one of the worst curses, irrespective of any wounds, remains the first and greatest sin: pride! Why not forget it, in these corridors of impersonal hospitals, which will not even notice its presence. What is certain is that cancer is stress. A divorce, a big failure, a failed childhood, are too. Nobody will avoid stress. I really like this statement by Boris Cyrulnik "... the worst stress is the absence of stress. Because lack of life before death, causes a desperate feeling of emptiness before emptiness."[13] The same Boris Cyrulnik, quotes in his book *A Wonderful Misfortune* the Romanian, Serge Moscovici (a child of totalitarianism): "I pity those who had a happy childhood, they have nothing to overcome"[14]. In this context, I will say something which I don't like! In fact, it won't please anyone. The best way to take a shortcut is to say, at the time of a painful shock, even and above all, if you do not think it: *Doxa To Theo*[15]! The Orthodox that I have visited in Greece and Cyprus repeat these three words at any moment. Joy, sorrow and trial. Yes, during trials ... great trials! *Glory to God*! I believe that it has happened to us all, the realisation, often years after a great misfortune, of the fruitfulness which it has brought to our souls! But this exclamation, which goes back to the first Christian martyrs, in no way dispenses with the fight. I will add that in these countries that I have mentioned, the faithful are accustomed to regular confession. It has nothing to do with the idiotic list of sins that are clever or less clever, and which must be played out in a mournful confessional. It is a matter of scrutinising, before

[13] Ibid, Page 36
[14] Ibid, Page 80
[15] Glory to God

God, before the icons and with the help of a *pneumatikos*[16], that which takes us away from God, and therefore from Life! Sin means that which is crooked, that which has missed its purpose! I'm losing focus and we'll talk about it, talk about it again and ... talk about it again! Because, if stress is unavoidable, no one is arguing today that chronic stress affects the immune system. Chronic means those old wounds that never stop getting sneakily reinfected. But also, these people around us, often close, who never finish "drinking our blood", according to an expression of my dear mother! Everyone can observe it in his or her life, becoming at one time or another "conscious" of it. This *pneumatikos* is none other than a priest who has received a sacramental blessing, to give the sacrament of forgiveness. This very old ecclesial custom allows for a very thorough and liberating dialogue. A relationship is established, which I personally compare, having practised both, to the relationship with one's therapist. Of course, the therapist did not receive the power of sacramental forgiveness! But sometimes, his or her training, openness, and listening, expand pastoral skills. If you don't support the idea of religion and still less the sacrament, then it would be a pity to deprive yourself of the extraordinary discoveries of modern psychology. Again, I repeat strongly: you're not married to your therapist. And before you make your big "transfer of affection", check if the person suits you. But as for the body, again, search, hit, move and ... dare!

Dare ...

Yes, dare, illness allows you to dare. Life, your family, your partner, your friends, your pride and your prejudices would never have dared. And then, the illness you have to overcome can receive a taste of complicity as well!

Melancholy, sadness, are often associated with somatic disease ... But can we dismiss them, under the pretext that we have cancer? It seems to me that all these past states or those that we come across, are a part of our life ... of me ... of you ... So start by not brooding, trying to chase regrets and what is

---

[16] The spiritual translation doesn't give the sense of the term.

worse: guilt!

A big burden, which gnaws insidiously, is passivity. Even though it is rooted, sometimes inherently so, in a state of chronic or genetic disease. Which, by the way, should hold us, once again, from any judgment upon others! But in a general way, it is watching us all. This apparent comfort that is gorged with tranquillity and immobility.

Immobility is death! I am thinking especially of the death of the soul. I met old monks, whose exhausted and worn-out bodies did not prevent their souls from being more alive than all the young souls that I could meet. In 2011, a few years before her death, I had the chance to meet Hélène Hoerni-Jung[17], the daughter of Carl Gustave Jung. A woman almost a hundred years old, who was moving with a walker. But thoughts walked with clarity in her head! We had tea ... over three hours. Both her vivacity, and her thirst for continuing to discover and transmit, remained for me, the sparkling life of the soul. Until an age more than canonical! This beautiful meeting was allowed to me, thanks to my friend Gabrielle. She was integrated within a small group of "faithful", who met regularly with this elder, for exchanges. Gabrielle, who lived through the earthquake in her infancy, had not only lost her father, but dealt with never knowing exactly when and where he had died. The latter, an Alsatian, enlisted by force, in the "malgré-eux", fell in Russia, during the second world war. Here is a beautiful example of resilience! Mother of three children, she strove with lucidity, never to parasitise them. She preferred to knock on the door of many analysts, including Marie-Louise von Franz[18]. Consciously, she is still fighting at age 83, in a perpetual quest, to create, communicate ... and grow! "We can transform ourselves at any time in our lives."[19] Still, we must want it ... to move ourselves... because, "Life is movement"[20]. Of course, this

---

[17] Hélène Hoerni-Jung (1914-2014), youngest daughter of Emma and Carl Jung, died in Küsnacht (Zürich) 1-07-2014. She had just celebrated her 100th birthday. Author of many works, among others upon Mary, the saints etc…

[18] Carl Gustave Jung's collaborator until his death.

[19] Dr. Frédéric Saldmann, *Votre Santé Sans Risque*.

[20] Ibid, page 14.

"movement" has nothing to do with the hysterical excitement of our modern world. Passing by everything, or almost ...

A few days ago I had the grace to converse with an old monk friend. I would like to ask a general and banal question, sparked by our dialogue: "What are we doing to feed our energies into a life-giving source?" Everyone must find their own answer, but the question deserves an answer. Faced with our failures, our discouragements, our diseases, our depression...

To return to more down-to-earth choices, here's what I try to put into practice in my daily life. I discipline myself to watch a maximum of two good movies per week. I choose them, according to my inner state, and their content must, first and foremost, please me. But I strive not to let the small screen eat up my energies, even if there are some excellent programmes. Instead, I work a few words of Greek, or I read, or I write. Similarly with my laptop, but here the fight is more difficult. I consult it, without it imposing its presence on me continuously. As if my being was welded to it, waiting for a message! Or news, which will not change anything in my life, if I discover it a little later. On the other hand, I try to remain awake, to all the little winks and nods of life ... that will enrich ... my belonging to *La Vie*. And I think meeting with the other, whoever he or she is, is a gift. I do not speak here only of parties, buffets: organised friend or family meetings become routine. I speak about the everyday, of what is unforeseen. Outside of the programme. There's this "crazy light", who I sometimes meet in the morning, in front of the home. He tells me his fantasies, the journeys he thinks he has made. His eyes are jet black, surrounded by black circles. No doubt he smokes too much. But when he laughs, and he laughs every time I talk to him, he manages to send me, from the depths of his night, the glittering star, that he managed to win from this shitty home! My heart communes ... At the moment of a laugh, our hearts commune ... What a slap to melancholy! To the anxieties, the misfortunes that may arise! The hospital ward or whatever else, can give you that desire for wonderment ... And, if it arises, then it must be preserved.

It is not a question of fleeing the reality of the internal struggle. Yes, if sickness or trials are triggered within you, this salutary reflex, then ... then ... this enemy will have been an accomplice. I think it starts with the desire to free oneself from established or imposed patterns. Religion; morality; fatalism; atheism; bigotry; clairvoyance; horoscopes; so-called freedoms; our brilliant intelligence and so on!

Yet it is a religious term, often repulsive, of which I will speak!

Of sin ...

Sin! Many millennia! I remember that since childhood I have been obsessed with sin. I wanted to know exactly what it was and I did not miss an opportunity to find out. The apple, the sex, the disobedience ... none of that satisfied my thirst for an answer. One day, before my conversion, at a conference given by an Orthodox priest, I did not fail to ask my favourite question: "And what exactly is sin?" I will never forget that frail little bearded man standing in front of me. He listened to my question, then he was silent for a long time. And he suddenly turned round. His back to the public. Always silent. After a few moments, he murmured: "That's what sin is: to turn your back on God ... to turn your back on Life!" I mentioned at the beginning of this book, "immature" parents who damage their children. We have all more or less been in this position! Because this blindness, this proud obstinacy to turn our backs on Life, on the laws of life, is repeated from generation to generation. Bringing with it the evils of the soul, but also the cosmic damage that we are now facing. And my illness, your illness, our illness is part of this "curse"! It starts with our internal or external escapism, our race to oblivion, into euphoria. Not to mention the tortures inflicted on the body by over-eating, drinking, narcotics, drugs, or disproportionate exhaustion. What an escalation! But as my Cypriot confessor recently said: "I was not born during the sin of Adam, how does it concern me?" Well, bigot, religious, atheist, liberated or otherwise, we drag with us, this sordid languor, that tar of the soul that gnaws at our vital energy! Do you think I'm exaggerating? Well tomorrow, decide to look for a psychotherapist who really puts you to work ... or a priest who listens to you in confession! You will see that it will never be without combat, without resistance! And yet neither you nor I have to bear the sin of Adam. Or ... if Adam does worry you, endure our imperfect nature, unfinished, as if it were a fatality! If there is a revolt that illness or an ordeal must bring, that's it! It opens a window onto rehabilitation. The restoration, or simply the beginning of an awareness that escapes this insolence of the unconscious and versatile child! This eternal *puer*[21], arrogant in his very emptiness, was he a great brain! Yes, I insist on this term! A great brain!

The Brain...

Sublime organ, except ... when it thinks it's a god!

Personally, I am fascinated by the discoveries of neurology and neuropsychiatry. Without alas understanding much, with my literary training! But what a horizon, what a universe! Blessed be these inspired brains who serve science. They shake up our shrunken visions! At the same time, I cannot bring myself to strike out the words "blessed" and "inspired". Neither can I fit them into the drawer of only chemical, physical or neurological reactions. Why does a sublime discovery, in turn, shrink the Infinite? As my Cypriot confessor often says: "God being infinite, we can never lock him in our brain!"

Hence, in the West, the damage caused by the distortions of scholasticism. In its efforts to explain what God and faith are. With the gradual erosion of the silence of prayer in the face of Mystery. But the modern scientific-spiritual scholasticism reduces the soul of man to these brilliant discoveries! How sad! Me, I sense a wink from God, collaborating with his creature. His creature, who by dint of humility (yes, it takes a lot of humility, to hang on to the search!) and hard work, is getting

---

[21] Child. Latin word.

closer and closer to His Creation ... Without ever quite drilling into the Mystery of the Encounter ... of Communion ... and ... of Love ...

As I encourage everyone, young and old, develop the brain by all means. But ... tame it a little too! Let it give way to the heart. Not to the denying and supposedly affectionate heart. No to the Heart that is able to enter into a relationship ... A relationship with the madman from the home, the rose in the garden, the tenderness of the night, or that of the morning mist ... but also ... with ...

The scent of mystery ...

Yes ... cross the border ... and enter into this Mystery that doesn't explain everything! At a conference organised by the neuropsychiatrist Boris Cyrulnik, in November 2013, one of the speakers, Professor Gérard Ostermann (internist and psychotherapist-analyst) said this sentence, made all the more beautiful by issuing from the mouth of a scientist: "There will never be a global theory of the psyche, nor will there be a global theory on the body, because it remains a mystery!" Theologians for their part (who are supposed to focus more on The Mystery and other mysteries) offer a picture so much more generous and authentic, when in turn they open the door to the discoveries of science. Integrating these discoveries without abandoning their faith and tradition. Once again, open, open, open and don't close the doors! This opening, which is the most sublime of the metamorphoses, is proposed to us all ... often ... yes ... often ... when sickness and trials arise. And in this sense, the enemy we are fighting against will also become an accomplice!

To "exploit" a little more the theme of sin, I want to quote Blessed Augustine[22], who speaking of the first sin, that of Adam and Eve, exclaims: "Happy fall, which earned us such a great redeemer!" We cannot go deeper into the ontology of being human. Whoever messed up ... messed up from the start.

[22] Augustin of Hippone (354-430)

Especially so, if this beginning is so timeless. Within the sublime Tradition of the Incarnation of the Son of God, entering into the flesh, the heart and the soul of man, offering him the freedom to metamorphose, the fall is, in fact, only a peccadillo, in the face of this "great redeemer"! However, this theology of the great Augustine, was often diverted to the West for the paralysing of souls, with this kind of feeling of there being in suffering some kind of fatal curse. I mentioned it at the beginning. As if you had to atone for sickness or some other misfortune! Conform to a distorted interpretation, that alone, the Son of God's mad act of love, satisfying God the Father's anger by his sacrifice on the cross, after the sins of his first creatures. Monstrous! As if God needed to be appeased. This twisted vision has no place in the Orthodox Tradition. Personally, I was completely unconsciously dragging around with me this "fatal punishment", facing an austere God, thirsting for appeasement. I insist: "totally unconsciously"! I was given the grace of finding a good analyst on my way. A good confessor also, in the pure Tradition of Love and Forgiveness. He was able to detect these underhanded deviations, that were torpedoing any intimate relationship with the Mystery of Communion with God. I hasten to add ... that yes, it was, it is, minute after minute, a long, very very long path! Including arriving at ... the therapist and the famous confessor!

The two biggest pitfalls are impatience and discouragement! Yes, your super diet does not bear immediate fruit. Yes, your physio monopolises your energies and you have the feeling of not advancing. Yes, you try to become more aware, more present, but the days pass and you fall back into your sticky routine!

Yes, you knock on doors and those which open themselves, are not the good ones! Hang on, do not despair! One of the greatest Athonite[23] saints was in the midst of his ascetic struggle in a terrible hell. Asking Christ to release him, he heard His answer: "Hold your soul in hell and do not despair!" Saint

---

[23] From Mont Athos in Greece.

Silouane then became one of the greatest contemporary saints (1866-1938).

May the reader forgive me these "planing" lines upon the spiritual life. In starting this book, I did not want to mention my faith. For reasons of comfort actually! Because, if we talk about organic food, yogic breaths, nature, or symbols and philosophy, it goes well. But if we put forward our faith in Christ, an essential component in all our battles, then we exclude and even annoy our public! But, faith is so much an integral part of my everyday life, that I could not leave it out. I have often mentioned the term "partnership". So here you are, the old madwoman you're reading, is always talking to her main partner ... and it's Christ! Christ, who spent his earthly life healing bodies and souls. Everyone will do what he or she wants. I shared this quest for "connection" as well, because this "connection" allowed me to go through suffering, heartbreak and illnesses ...

Not any better than anyone else ... absolutely not!

Absolutely not...

Nor in a superior or extraordinary way! But ... it's my course...

I return to basic (more down to earth!) help that I will never repeat enough, even if it seems obvious. It is to start the day with something very banal: breathing ... but ... breathe consciously. Not necessarily great yogic feats. Simply feel that you are breathing and if possible, with a little or a lot of fresh air. Me, I close a nostril with my finger, I breathe in, then exhale and do the same thing with the other. At each breath, I pray. A prayer about life ... or a prayer for my doctors ... my relatives ... those who have fallen asleep. Do you not pray? And send good thoughts to others ... or send that breath to your sick body! You will find what suits you. And you will see, this meeting with your breath, with The Breath will become an ally. You will not be able to do without it. Start with five breaths, then increase it a little.

This routine only takes about ten minutes. But it mustn't be confused with precise, therapeutic breathing, for asthma, for example, or to strengthen the muscles in the spine.

It's an appointment with awakening ...

With ... the presence of life!

You can also ... imagine your angel, your guardian angel. As we saw them in old children's books ... and ask each breath to strengthen you, to guide you, to protect you ...

Accept being guided by something other than nothing ...

Other ... than ... nothing!

We breathe better, if we focus on something. Especially since the mind often wanders and ends up spoiling it - and this is not only true when one has cancer.

As soon as the storm of surgeries and major treatments has passed, we must continue to strengthen this Heart that has been stripped bare ...

I will express the platitude that cancer, often associated with death, will have given you an advantage. It is precisely that you are mortal. Yes, yes ...

I need to open a parenthesis, for a lovely story told to me by a friend, a Cypriot priest:

In the village there was a magnificent old man. Strong and robust. Not only had he never been ill, but he kept saying: "I will never be sick, besides I will not die, I will never die!" One day, when he was sitting, as usual at his door, he saw an adorable little boy arrive. Dressed in a small sailor suit, with a white shirt and a bow tie. The little boy was sucking on a lollipop. As children his age often do. The old man rejoiced immensely at the sight of this little boy whom he did not know. He called him to him and asked him happily, "Hello, my dear, what are you doing here?" Then the little boy answered him: "I am finishing my lollipop ... and then poof! ... off we go, it's time for you!"

At least your cancer, your hepatitis or any other serious illness, brings you awareness that this time will come sooner or later. It's not about becoming morbid, no, no! But this "poof ... and off we go!" has been present, from the first moment of the medical verdict ... So, put another slant on life, on your life ... At the moment, as I write these lines, the blackbirds are singing, as they do every day at this hour. Have you noticed, a thing so beautiful, a blackbird who sings ... who sings for free?

I also like to hold a pebble in my hand ... How long has it been rolling in torrents, in the sea, on the roads? Our lives of 10, 30, 60 or 90 years, what are they, in the face of eternity? A spark ... So this spark is as bright as possible!

And then, it's time to protect your heart. You are not here to judge the world under the pretext that you have had, or are going through, a cancer or a terrible ordeal. But you are no longer there, to meet up with those who bring the worst out in you! Because we all have this, the worst in us ... It's time to look for the people who bring the best out of you. The best of your heart ... the best of your life ... the best of your smile ... the best of your laugh!

Laugh as often as possible ... a sublime therapy!

Practice also making choices, knowing that you cannot do everything! Know it then, recognise your priorities!

Another effective therapy, that is often meaningless in a world where "thank you" is rarely said, is recognition. Express gratitude, for care, for forgiveness, for life! Scientists say that a sustained feeling of gratefulness extends the life span.

Thus, by consciously weeding people out, choosing disciples of life and not the deadly grunts, by sorting images and everything, what then enters your heart will lead you to a joyful serenity. This serenity will not steer you clear of other moments of suffering, but with your cancer, your test, you will start to rebuild yourself in the valley of shadows ... Rebuild yourself ... By accepting that you fall, that you're weak, that you're wrong, that you're wading about... and that you are starting again ... to fight ... to live ...

To live there, where a communion with light becomes a true hope ...

Neither must one be fearful about scrutinising their soul, the possible traps, both conscious and above all unconscious, of the "benefits" of the disease. They are insidious. Without going into the generalities of first-degree psychology, everyone should ask themselves the question, what message is being expressed through their body? Or even ... what are they gaining from their condition? And then make sure that the disease does not become an hostile accomplice.

I open a parenthesis, I am about to use a religious phrase that has a very bad reputation: penitence! In Greek, the word is *metanoia*. The best translation that I have heard recently was from an old Cypriot Priest Monk: *"change of noûs"*. The *noûs*[24] corresponds to the most intimate heart of man. In French, we would translate *metanoia* with the word *pénitence*, which is a word that has been subject to much derision over the centuries!

In the traditional way of seeing it, the most effective penitence consists in seeing oneself as one really is.

Stop keeping up that continual pretence!

To recognise oneself, mad or less mad, with faults, failings, hidden desires. The most moving symbol of this state, remains that of the first to enter The Kingdom: the good thief! He who was crucified with Christ. He knew how to recognise his condition and, at the same time, the innocence of Him who was crucified with him. Parenthesis: good morals, take a hit! The first in paradise with Christ, is none other than a ... bandit ... But ... a bandit who recognised himself as such! So, try to enter this kingdom of liberation, which is the refusal to engage in hypocrisy about yourself! Free yourself, at the same time, from the judgment and the gaze of others, who push you to do that which you often do not want to do! And when you do something, do it with your whole being and your entire commitment!

I like this "asceticism" of a friend, a Greek Priest Monk, who applies it, more precisely to "salvation". But ... your salvation and your health begin here, at this very moment:

Three essential points:

---

[24] No suitable French or English equivalent!

1. Give your body what it needs, otherwise it will claim it.
2. Always be as conscious as possible, present in what you do.
3. Through everything that happens to you, keep Christ in your heart!

If this last point doesn't correspond with your beliefs, you do however know that Christ has loved and forgiven. Well, offer to your heart love and forgiveness, as images of gratitude and life. Above all, if you cannot apply them, do not worry, me neither! But they are universal, eternal forces and they can only bring to you a little peace, communion and ... energy.

You will not be bigoted! What do you have to lose?

In a very concrete sense, I come back to the second point. Conscious presence often evaporates in routine. Yes, daily constancy must become your best ally. But beware of it changing into an insidious enemy. In unfeeling and unhearing habits, with which you perform your exercises, your breaths, your prayers, sometimes at speed. And even, with which you look at those you love ...

Nothing…

Nothing is ever acquired, for staying alive!

So, we must agree to stop or put on the brakes a little ... Quantity must never engulf quality. According to this beautiful quote by Oscar Wilde: "We must not seek to add years to our life, but rather try to add life to our years."

Take care of your body, your soul, your heart, without feeling the centre of the world. Neither ignore that others are suffering, right now. So you, who have gone through hell, offer your smile, whenever possible. It is also a way of being grateful, which can only enrich you with positive waves. I would add finally, that nobody is obliged to let themselves be swallowed up by the most negative news. Neither by biographies that dish the dirt ... In contrast, favour the permanent return, to Mother Nature. With her secrets, her treasures, her fertile silences and her inexhaustible heritage of wisdom.

I would also like to point out some pitfalls:

Above all, becoming obsessed with Holy Health! Avoiding

the slightest risk, which amounts to killing off Life. Forgetting that we will never control everything! Also, I give myself one "joker" day a week. In general, a Sunday. Rest! No physio, no food vigilance, without however rushing into any gargantuan orgies.

Which brings us to the trap of comparing our own plate to that of the "happy Gargantua". I often lamented in airplanes, my neighbours' omelettes, sausages, alcohol and sweets!

And also ... don't be discouraged, if the mastery of our more selective lifestyle makes us paradoxically more delicate. Obviously, the body is not crazy and it is alarmed at the first disturbances. The soul too! This may be all the more upsetting, if part of our social fabric is critical of what we call our "rebirth"! It must be known that those who have never been in a state of severe illness or a hardship are rarely able to understand ...

Another obstacle, I repeat, is that the results are not immediate! You must keep trying. But, you'll see, you will feel better, not only in your body, but also in your soul!

This "Rebirth"

IT IS OBVIOUS THAT one cannot change one's life, one's behaviours (relational, psychological or nutritional) with a snap of the fingers! But if there is a benefit to be gained from suffering, it is that of having consciousness. And in many areas at that. Just in citing those of human relations, we will realise what we already knew. It is certain that one has more "friends", if one has a villa on the Riviera, than if one is at the bottom of a hospital bed, or in a home! Nothing new under the sun, but this awareness must be managed. The pitfalls to avoid are rancour or even despair. This is perhaps the moment to draw vitality from these mutations, whatever they are. Anyway, you have rubbed up against death, why would you risk more?

I have experienced that we meet new friends at any age. And the links are even stronger, since it makes sense to know your own heart a little better! Finally, learn that "no" is also a respectable word! And if you have to banish all judgment, the most sterile feeling that there is, you can choose to enter finally into communion with people who wish for it as much as you. What is more precious than a communion, without make-up, parade, lost points or points to score against the others?

If I respect certain obligations, and avoid hurting my moments of communion, I choose to share them with those who are ready to share. And if there is no one around, there will always be a blackbird, a gull, a raven, a robin or a big crab that will do the trick! It is said that one of Louis XIV's famous prisoners, Academician Pelisson, astonished the director of the Bastille by his sudden change of mood. In fact, in his prison he had managed to tame ... a big spider! I repeat it insistently, it is not a question of selecting geniuses, nor of becoming a misogynist, but we will always have a need of others. Even the hermits of Athos leave to retire to a little isolated community, with the agreement of their spiritual father. Often, they return on a Sunday, for communal work with the brothers, that of the liturgy. Simply, I try as much as possible, not to waste the life I was left with, to participate in a social masquerade, or even a family one. But again, this is not a value judgment. These are paths that will never meet ... or never again. On this subject, I like to remember a phrase repeated by one of my old theology professors: "We are not responsible for what others think of us, but we are responsible for what the we think of others!"

Yes ... yes, we must become responsible for what we think! For me, it means to consciously distance myself from that which damages my heart. What energy gained ... but what an asceticism! What an immense, eternal asceticism!

Because our heart is constantly besieged, beginning with ... our own bullshit!

Asceticism, the word is dropped! It doesn't mean anything other than "exercise".

Whatever the changes in your relationships, your way of life, your thoughts, your way of nourishing your body and your soul, you must know that it is an intense fight, but also an exciting one! As in any fight, there will be chaos, failures, relapses, discouragements, annoyances! I'm crossing them all! But what is great is that you are alive and you will become so more and more! So, get up, start again, sob your heart out or laugh, but go on ... go on ... go on! "Success is not final, failure is not fatal: it is the courage to continue that counts."[25]

The courage to continue ...

I believe that the humiliations of sickness and hardships are a big slap in the face to your well-modelled image or ... sometimes ... *de*-modelled by your surroundings. It may well be the opportunity then, to go in search of your true image! More ...

[25] Churchill.

authentic ... more intimate ...

Remember that communion!

Communion with the food you choose, enjoy, chew. With the air you breathe, that you will breathe again. With the images you want to keep. With nature. With your body. With your heart. With the hearts of those who share with you. However, this communion has nothing to do with seduction. In all its forms. Erotic, intellectual, psychic or ... of doubtful spirituality! And I push the pawn even further, at the risk of shocking:

The true, authentic communion in all relationships is attained only in ... the Holy Spirit, "... Comforter, Spirit of truth ..."[26]

What a struggle, yes ... to know, who you really are ... and to commune with these others who are so different, but at the same time so close, in this sublime conquest of the authenticity of presence.

And then ... if the disease has stayed and remains an enemy for me, I keep using the term "accomplice". Just like the ordeal, it brought me the courage to express myself, without fear, of not being loved, or admired! Which allows me to add this reflection:

I am convinced that this part of our soul that we call "the unconscious", in using old or recent wounds, is eating away at our vital energy. And even if it displeases some religious people, modern psychotherapeutic science is one of the rare keys, to excavate these wounds from the shade. In order to stop them already in their sly suppuration. But no offence to some "scientists of the soul", just the fact of removing these wounds is not enough for complete healing!

And, that's where Christ comes in ... and forgiveness ...

Forgive me, "For the evil that I do and the good that I do not do."[27]

Especially ... especially ... to feel, to know ... I'm forgiven ...

To know myself forgiven ... what a beautiful skylight onto the Kingdom ...

---

[26] Orthodox prayer to the Holy Spirit.
[27] Letter to the Romans 7:19

But also ... to forgive ...

To forgive ... or rather ... to start forcing myself to pray, for those who have hurt me, or who have torn apart so much, those whom I loved ...

I am obliged, for my testimony to be more complete, to specify two things:

First of all, what a joy to reconnect with writing! The illness pushed me towards this new project, to find the passion that has lived in me since adolescence! With an unexpected therapeutic aspect! In this book, I became aware of a "trauma" related to "no right to life!" From ... the maternal womb ... revealed, by the banal question of a child. Psychotherapy had already tracked this process, the writing validates it. Yes ... some "tolls" are also related to this shock that has resurfaced through my story ... So, I encourage you, dig into yourself and discover what is buried ... and most importantly, what you want to achieve! It's never ... never ... never too late!

Finally ... the discovery of life, in the face of Christ, without judgment or morality has helped me and helps me, as I just said.

It's up to you to search ... to seek out finally, without any prejudice, what will guide you ...

I cannot help but mention again this phase of a great Cypriot saint that I venerate. Saint Neophyte:

"The good above all good is the fear of God and the memory of death."

With that, she breaks apart old age!

She pulls us apart completely! First, she gives us health advice, battle plans against the enemy disease. Then she tells us that she has faith in a Christ who neither judges nor moralises ... but forgives. To conclude with the fury of God and the memory of death!

That's my explanation:

The fear of God, in the original Tradition, is acceptance before the Mystery! Accept that you will never know or control your life, or even what you think you know about yourself. It is the sacred fear, in front of this setting sun, or in a beauty that takes your breath away. This moon, which rises with a tenderness that tears you away! It is this place of pilgrimage, oozing the sacred. This radiant look of fire that yet is flooded with peace ... It is to accept that, whatever you do, there will always be an unforeseen, a suffering, a joy, a desire, a door that will open at the moment when you did not expect more ... Or ...

Or...

Or...

One day...

Inevitably, for each of us, the door ... which will close ...

Close to life, life on earth anyway.

So, do not be morbid, but remember that ...

Death is ... still ... a little ... our little sister!

And ... maybe we have to prepare too, to meet her ...

It will only make you more fearless, to ... catch up with your life ...

I want to report Dad's last words, who returned to his atheism, just up until the end of his life. It was, as if he had received at the time of departure, a "new vision":

"Basically, it will be a jump, a trip ... and ..." His face was illuminated: "And ... we will all meet again!"

Mum, she had a strange reaction, but it was just as moving:

Her face was transfigured, she looked to the end of the empty room and whispered to me with a magnificent smile: "Oh ... I saw ... I saw ... I see ..."

I like to think that she saw the only love of her life, who came looking for her ...

A life of communion, with an immense, unique love!

In my arms died successively, in the space of three years, my father, my mother and my only brother. While I can admire these old images of a time where the dying were surrounded by their family, today, the beds of the dying frighten people more and more. Of course, there is no more painful a cut than that of receiving the last sigh of a loved one. But if, in defiance of your strength (yes, there are sacred exceptions to your lifestyle!) and your fragile health, you have accompanied them with your presence and your love, so ... these last moments are ... blessed... They will give you an inner strength, that no one else, nor anything else, will take away from you. If you can, do not hide ...

It's not a matter of getting it over with quickly, of gleaning that experience of the last sigh, of something to show off about during your soirées, neither is it to scare you, nor to show that you are not afraid.

Or even reassure you, whether you are a Christian or a philanthropist ...

No, this is about your blood. That of your exhausted flesh ... Nothing is more exhausting than to accompany another's suffering, with a quartered heart ...

Once again, everyone reacts differently. However, I would like to insist again. On the necessity of the antinomy. Do not fall into the "either / or" ... Hang on to "and / and"! Sometimes you have to know how to tame the opposites ... An art that can only enrich. Once again, traditional theology is a leaven of flexibility of mind about it! Accept God and Man at the same time! Virginity and motherhood ... Accept that two opposites are fertile! Thus, it is essential to protect your body and your vital organs, because we can do nothing here below without our body! But it is just as vital, to maintain a balance, which sometimes consists of engaging oneself, and getting exhausted! To no longer spare oneself at all, in order to live... that which must still be experienced. Also remember, that anyway, the body will wear out and that it will not go into eternity, at least not this way! No, you will not erase the curse of death, so be discerning about the living you can still do ... so that your heart and your soul grow ... And, why not? ... lead you to the limits of reason ...

Over there...

All over there ... where ... you may be able, at the hour, to whisper:

"I saw ... I ... see ..."

When Carl Jung was asked if he believed in God, he said, "I

do not believe, I know!"[28]

To leave, to leave again ... and to leave again, in search of these wells ... to water our energies.

To a life-giving source ... to a Source ...

Vivified ...

To dare to be dragged towards the love ...

This Love, which offers us infinitely, the sublime and perilous freedom ... that of limiting us, of suffocating ourselves ... by turning our back on Him!

Uniqueness.

Communion.

Lightness too ...

The one that invites butterflies into my soul ...

For an enchanted waltz ...

A healthy food that makes me light (well almost!)

Humour about my own little "case... case"... in the immensity of eternity...

A smile…

A laugh, whenever possible ...

A laugh that does not make fun of anything ...

No, a laugh that loves ...

Complicity with any form of life ...

With ... lives, your life, our lives ...

If we accept what sin represents, that which turns our backs on life, that which has missed its target, or which is twisted. So this question of Christ's to the paralysed man is addressed to each one of us:

"Do you want to be healed?"[29]

Do you ... want ... to be healed?

Under the jealous and critical gaze of hypocrites, the paralysed man stands up and walks ... Christ, then, will say to him:

"Go and sin no more ..."[30]

---

[28] Interview of Carl Gustave Jung with John Freeman, BBC, October 1959
[29] John 5, 1-6
[30] John 5, 1-6

Sin no more ...
Do not turn ... your back on life!
Do not turn your back ... on your life!
Do not turn your back ...
on The Life...

Biel, July 1, 2018
*Feast of The Holy Anargyrous of
Rome, Come and Damien.*

POSTSCRIPT
– OCTOBER 2022

COVID-19

That which in my book *The Tenth Plague*[31] I call "Minus" ended up ensnaring me after almost three years of being cautious...

Fortunately he waited, because the 2022 variants are less virulent, and fortunately I had received three doses of vaccines. As everyone can guess, I would have preferred not to write this postscript, but I am taking it as an opportunity to list what has helped me. Again these are only personal experiences which should be verified with a qualified medical professional for each unique case.

Prevention:

As far as I'm concerned I would prioritise the vaccines that leave traces of antibodies. I will take my fourth dose (according to the guidance) four months after the start of my infection which, in principle, has created new antibodies.

But as my friend, Professor Denis Malvy from Bordeaux[32], humbly told me, "medicine remains an imprecise science". This should encourage us to be tentative in our response rather than launch into sterile polemics.

Finally, the mundane action of washing and sanitising hands with disinfectant and wearing the FFP2 mask in places where you are at risk.

The progress of my infection:

One morning, I was hit with the famous exhaustion that is so heavy that it hurts! In the afternoon I went to the pharmacy for an antigen test which

---

[31] Maria Andreas, Revised Edition Amazon 2022

[32] Doctor and epidemiologist, member of the scientific council during lockdown.

turned out to be negative. Coming back, I walked with difficulty, as out of breath as ever. At night I shivered and I coughed (a rather dry cough) continuously. The next day, headaches, body aches, weakness and coughing. On the third day, I did a PCR test which is positive. It is the most accurate test.

Two painful weeks followed. If the aches and headaches disappear quickly, diarrhea sets in; my already present gastric problems worsen and the cough persists. A still rather dry and painful symptom that clings on. A kind of ball in the throat and on the bronchi that sticks in a mass, very difficult to transform into mucus and spit out. At the end of the third week, thanks to the inhaled cortisone treatment, this ball diminishes and only a sporadic cough persists.

The fever never high, even low at first, then around 38 C, returns to normal after a few days. Exhaustion gives way to great fatigue, that of a struggling body.

My treatments:
It is well known that except for its infectious complications, there are no treatments for this virus. However, Professor Denis Malvy[33] recommended Paxlovid to me, given my medical pedigree. An antiviral which to be effective must be taken from the first days. I did not find this in my provincial Swiss town where no one had even heard of it! I think I had an excellent reaction, that of not panicking and telling myself that I was going to fight without this antiviral.

I then stuck to the following medications:

Paracetamol to relieve pain.
Acetylcysteineum 600 mg (Flumicil / Solmucol or other) to liquefy and evacuate mucus. 1 effervescent tablet after breakfast.
Same effect but plant-based GeloDurat (1 tablet morning / noon and / evening at bedtime)
Bronchipret tablets or syrup, always in phytotherapy
In homeopathy: Arsenicum 15 CH or Bryonia 15 CH
I didn't take anything for the diarrhoea except brewer's yeast supplements with zinc.
Vitamin D too, known to help against Covid.
As for my stomach on fire, I started a 15mg Lansoprazol remedy, 1 tablet in the evening, 1 tablet in the morning 30 minutes before eating. But as already mentioned, these disorders which worsened with Covid were already preexisting.
In the evening, when going to bed I also took a tablet of Digebiane (Pileje

---

lab), a food supplement recommended by my homeopath.

Continuous thyme herbal teas.

Hot water.

A little eucalyptus honey to which I add a pinch of turmeric.

In the morning on an empty stomach (and this can also be taken as a prophylactic): a teaspoon of olive oil with a pinch of turmeric (beware of its anticoagulant effect in high doses) and clove powder.

Vitamin C Acerola in the morning.

Lozenges of all kinds (avoid sugar) to moisten the throat or soothe irritation. In the latter case, my favourites are based on propolis. (Also available in sprays).

Eucalyptus essential oil inhalations.

In the evening, a few drops of Ravintsara essential oil to massage on the wrists.

And then, alas, in my case of bronchi weakened by an asthmatic background, I had to repeat a course of inhaled cortisone after two weeks as – what do you think – the cough was still around! (Only on medical prescription and with the doctor's agreement). Revlar Ellipta 92/22mg. By the third dose, the symptoms of a lump stuck in the throat and the choking cough improved. If you have to take it, I recommend rinsing your mouth, even cleaning your teeth, after inhalation. This is to avoid possible minor inflammations of the mouth. Personally, I do my inhalation just before breakfast.

During non-stop coughing and insomnia, I tested two drops of CBD (cannabidiol 20%). I hated the taste but it had the positive effect of relaxing me a bit so I had a better chance of resting during the big crisis.

Three weeks on, I have just resumed my respiratory therapy which consists of blowing as hard and for as long as possible into a small device adapted to this kind of exercise. (It costs only a few euros). I will resume my yogic breathing when the cough no longer interrupts it. As soon as it became possible, I started walking again, trying to maintain the balance which consists in not exhausting the body, while finding a rhythm.

Psychological battle

As I wrote in the October 26, 2022 postscript to my book, *The Tenth Plague*, I felt "like a piece of old shit." No other choice than to draw on your reserves whatever they are. Having lost eight acquaintances (from 42 to 95 years old) during the first two years of the pandemic, I went through moments of anguish that neither prayer, nor relaxation, nor anything at all could appease. But I continued to eat well, to drink a lot. At the first signs of inflammation, however, I eliminated dairy products and I even replaced my butter with white marzipan.

In this phase of disorientation, I was helped by the support of my (thank God spared) friend's daily telephones. But also by the "anti-depression basket" that my niece left for me at the front door, with, among other things, a huge portion of artfully cooked pumpkin soup. Also, if you are not sick but know relatives or less close relatives who are sick, don't hesitate to do a good deed! Each little message is also a balm when we are wading through the night. And then, the everyday but beneficial distraction of a good movie, because reading is difficult at the heart of the crisis. As soon as my strength returned, I rushed to my favourite therapy, the one that saves me every time: writing. Thus, I have completed my children's tale: *I Tell You Never Give Up*[34], a postscript for *The Tenth Plague* and those lines which the reader has just discovered.

It is still not an ordinary virus that we sometimes talk about lightly. Especially when you are not infected or when you are in good enough health to resist it!

Even in its less virulent form, it takes energy to overcome it, and at the end of the third week, I am continuing to fight. But once again, the ability to react is incredible, enriched by a new bad experience!

So I believe that no one will be able to escape this momentum which remains one of the most beautiful that man can feel...

Gratitude.

Gratitude for the most precious gift:

Life...

The one that makes an old fool dream that a valiant warlord will agree to sit down with a tyrant, however monstrous that tyrant might be. So that the people he loves have a chance, even the smallest chance, to live and escape martyrdom.

Or quite simply...the one who accepts that the other has not gone through the disease in the same way as me and does not consider it a major enemy.

Gratitude though...

Because, whatever the size of our spirit, "the body", as Saint Seraphim of Sarov[35] said, remains our "best friend"...

---

[34] To be published next
[35] Russian saint (1754-1883)

Bibliography

David Servan-Schreiber, *Anticancer,* Pocket.

Pr David Khayat, *Le Vrai régime anticancer*, Odile Jacob.

Dr Richard Béliveau & Denis Gingras, *La méthode anticancer*, J'ai lu.

Dr Denis Gingras & Dr Richard Béliveau, *Les aliments contre le cancer*, Solar.

Anna Le Marchand, *Chouchoutez votre cerveau*, Rustica.

Dr Frédéric Saldmann, *Le meilleur médicament, c'est vous !* Le livre de poche.

Dr Frédéric Saldmann, *Votre santé sans risque*, Albin Michel.

Dr Frédéric Saldmann, *Prenez votre santé en main* ! Albin Michel

Pr. Henri Joyeux & Jean Joyeux, *Manger mieux et meilleur*, Ed du Rocher

Henri Joyeux, *Guérir enfin du cancer*, Ed du Rocher

Boris Cyrulnik, *Un merveilleux malheur*, Odile Jacob

By the Same Author

Arthritis, Osteoporosis, Breast cancer and Other
Scourges – Amazon, 2019
Sparkles of Intensity – Amazon, 2020
The Tenth Plague – Huge Jam, 2021
Raphaela's 24-Hour Detox - Huge Jam, 2021
Cyprus, Your Heart, Your History – Amazon, 2022
Hook Up with Your Angel – Huge Jam, 2022
Cyprus I Have Embraced Your Heart - Hgfe Jam, 2022

Be the first to know about new books
by signing up to the newsletter at
www.mariaandreas.eu.

Would you recommend this book? Please leave
reviews on Amazon and Goodreads to help the author
extend her readership...

About the Author

<www.mariaandreas.eu>

MARIA ANDREAS WAS BORN in Algiers in 1950, of French-Swiss nationality. In the 70s, leftist and antimilitarist, she obtained her Baccalaureate at *La Chaux-de-Fonds*. She began her literary studies in Neuchâtel, then in Zürich, where she graduated from secondary school. She embarked then, following the hippie tradition of the time, aboard a small camper van, for a long trip in Asia, then in North Africa. She was fascinated by Buddhism and any new culture. She then worked in London, and Cambridge where she obtained her teaching qualification. For 25 years, she taught French literature at the *Dr.Pfister Institute* in Oberägeri, in German-speaking Switzerland. She learnt her profession, but also the democratic and Christian tradition of Switzerland. It is illness that compels her to leave her students. Based in Bordeaux, she devoted herself to distance learning. She obtained a Bachelor's degree in Theology at the *Saint-Denys Institute* in Paris, a certificate of study at the *Saint-Serge Institute of Theology* in Paris and a certificate in Applied Psychology at the *LAPP Institute* in Dusseldorf. Following a long Jungian analysis, trials and sickness projected her to the Byzantine world. She fell in love with the spirituality of the traditional Orthodox monasteries, the Greek language and stayed for a year in Cyprus. She then decided to reconnect with her writing, for which she had already won first prize for her dissertation in the *European Schools Competition of Strasbourg* in 1967.

www.ingramcontent.com/pod-product-compliance
Lightning Source LLC
Chambersburg PA
CBHW061505250726
48657CB00005B/1728